slow beauty

rituals and recipes to nourish the body and feed the soul

SHEL PINK

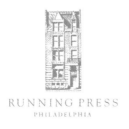

RUNNING PRESS
PHILADELPHIA

Running Press
Hachette Book Group
1290 Avenue of the Americas, New York, NY 10104
www.runningpress.com
@Running_Press

Printed in China

First Edition: November 2017

Published by Running Press, an imprint of Perseus Books, LLC,
a subsidiary of Hachette Book Group, Inc.

The Hachette Speakers Bureau provides a wide range of
authors for speaking events. To find out more, go to
www.hachettespeakersbureau.com or call (866) 376-6591.

The publisher is not responsible for websites (or their content) that are not
owned by the publisher.

Photography by Marissa Berrini

Cover photograph by Jovana Rikalo / Stocksy.com

Illustrations on pages 88, 90, 179, 192, 207, 208, 209, 210 by Christina
Bautista. Illustrations on pages 16 and 170 by Jameela Wahlgren

Print book cover and interior design by Susan Van Horn.

Library of Congress Control Number: 2017945838

ISBNs: 978-0-7624-6256-8 (paperback), 978-0-7624-6257-5 (ebook)

RRD-S

10 9 8 7 6 5 4 3 2 1

This book is dedicated to all the women who do, and ever will, live and love on this planet, and to those who came before us. Onward!

Contents

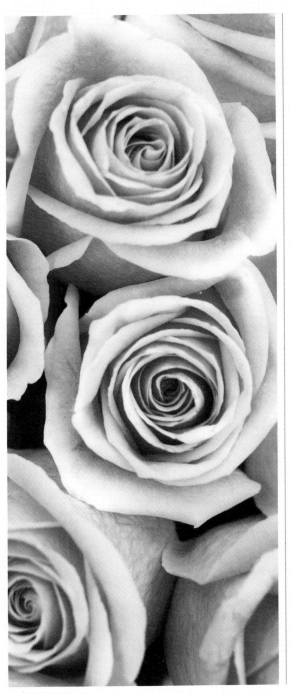

about
SLOW
BEAUTY

HOW MANY TIMES HAVE YOU HEARD some version of the phrase *beauty comes from within*? My guess is that the answer to this question is something along the lines of "a lot." Yet, at the same time, social media, magazines, and even newspapers are constantly flooding us with information about antiaging methods, and tips and tricks for enhancing our external beauty. If beauty comes from within, then where is all of this advice and strategy for illuminating our inner beauty?

Well, here it is.

The Slow Beauty practice that you are about to embark upon has nothing to do with creating the perfect smoky eye or combating wrinkles. Instead, it's about living a life that centers on a philosophy of living better, more wholly, and more truthfully—and having fun in the process! That is where true beauty springs forth: bubbling up from the inside and spilling over to the outside. At the heart of the Slow Beauty philosophy and practice is the idea that the biggest component of any beauty program should be wellness and self-care. To achieve this, we must each regularly find some time to slow down and connect with ourself.

Within the pages that follow, you'll find inspiration, support, and tools for cultivating that beauty within to the point where it spills over to every aspect of your life, including your physical appearance. Yes, we'll talk about beauty, but we'll also focus on general wellness, aging happily and gracefully, and—most important of all—cultivating a truly *joyful* life from the inside out.

Know that this practice is called *Slow* Beauty for a reason. It's what I like to think of as a *sustainable* beauty alternative. It's not a quick fix—much better than that, it's a solution that will last over time. It will become an inextricable part of your life. And, as I've seen in both my own life and the lives of the clients I've worked with, the ongoing journey of Slow Beauty will be one of the most fulfilling, adventurous, creative, and transformative experiences you've ever embarked upon. Rather than a chore or source of stress, this ongoing beauty routine will become a cherished part of your day-to-day life.

Slow Beauty marks a return to our connection with our personal natural rhythms, and ultimately, it brings us back to an unconditional love and acceptance of becoming who we really are. When we live in this sort of manner over a period of time, we naturally and continuously evolve into a more beautiful and timeless version of ourself. Most of all, we find more joy in our life on a moment-by-moment basis. And that is truly beautiful.

Together, we'll get in touch with the type of beauty that starts from within and emanates outward from there. The type of beauty that defies age. The type of beauty that knows no bounds.

the four pillars of slow beauty

Slow Beauty encapsulates such ideals as inner beauty, self-love, self-care, self-compassion, and joyful living in what is less of a program, and more of an open-source system that will make you look and feel better. This is *not* a prescriptive program, although I definitely will share tons of ideas for you to incorporate into your own life. Like the Slow Beauty program itself, this book is meant to be playful, iterative, and interactive. With that in mind, there are many ways to enjoy it. There is, of course, the traditional approach of reading it from cover to cover and trying everything in the order in which it is presented. Another option is to engage with it in whatever way feels most natural to you. For example, if you are feeling active, begin with a ritual or a recipe. If you feel as if you need some intellectual stimulation, dive into the Philosophy section. Ready to get creative? Flip to the Mapping section.

With this in mind, Slow Beauty is divided into four distinct sections—the Four Pillars of Slow Beauty, if you will.

PHILOSOPHY

What kind of beauty book starts with *philosophy* of all things, right? At a glance, it might sound a bit odd to correlate beauty and philosophy. But Slow Beauty is all about an elevated type of beauty that comes from the inside and, from there, takes up residency in all aspects of our life. Since Slow Beauty is also, in many ways, a personal program that each of us determines the specifics of ourself, it's important that it be built upon a foundation and a framework people can understand, get behind, and incorporate into their daily life.

There was a time when philosophy was not only the cornerstone of education, but also of life in general. People had an underlying ethos that informed many facets of their life: the way they thought, what they believed in, and the decisions they made on a moment-by-moment basis.

Over time, philosophy has become a less and less integral part of our system and our life. Look at any college curriculum today and you'll see a vast difference in how much philosophy is introduced to students, even between now and a couple of decades ago. Our society's concept of philosophy is now doled out in little nuggets through articles shared on Facebook and Instagram memes. Something may resonate with us, but it is fleeting, and before long, we've moved on to the next thing. Most of us don't have a solid credo to hold on to.

We live in a world that moves quickly, and we're constantly pulled in different directions. So many of us are wearing this stress; we don't feel good because of it, and when we don't feel good, we don't look good, either. It's time to slow down and get back in touch with life and ourself. The Slow Beauty philosophy provides us with a touchstone to do that through its belief that it is by making the time to go inward to discover what lights us up and bring us joy—and then honoring that—that we ultimately find true, lasting, timeless beauty. It gives us ideas to marinate on and take with us, and allows these seeds of self-care to continue to grow, even amid all the white noise of our life.

Beauty is multifaceted and inherently simultaneously spiritual and biological. If we care for ourself in deep and meaningful ways, then we are better able to care for others and for the world around us. If we want to slow down, enjoy life, and be well, the Slow Beauty philosophy will help us to discern, engage, and amplify what is a most true and creative process—being our most beautiful, healthy self!

So, how will we know this is working for us? How will we be able to celebrate how we are changing? Or even know we are on the right path? First we need to acknowledge the "new normal": the frantic, nonstop pace of our life today. We shouldn't have to merely accept and adapt to this new pace of life. This isn't about continuing at this insane pace, it's about *challenging* that pace. It's about finding our *own* pace and grounding ourself in it. It's a question of pace for inner peace, and from that slower pace the seeds of enlightenment are planted. At the core of the Slow Beauty philosophy is discovering ways to slow down, because it is only then that renewal happens.

RITUALS

One of the primary ways we put the Slow Beauty philosophy into practice is through rituals. As Princeton sociologist Robert Wuthnow put it, we are currently living in the Age of Practice. He explains, "In the United States, religious life has evolved from a 'dwelling spirituality' in the 1950s, when the physical church or synagogue building was the focus of family religious life; to a

'seeking spirituality' of the turbulent 1960s, when the individual's quest for personal meaning and moments of transcendence stood at the center; to our age—an age of meditation practice communities and yoga practice communities."

Wuthnow points to this trend in an academic sense, but you've most likely already noticed it at play in your own life. Maybe you practice yoga yourself; if not, you likely know many others who do or have noticed its increasing prominence in society. The ancient practice of meditation is now becoming mainstream in the same way yoga has in the past decade.

So, what does all of that have to do with Slow Beauty? Slow Beauty is something to be practiced, and a big part of this practice includes meditative techniques, both in the traditional sense and in the terms of rituals that can be meditative in nature when practiced mindfully. *Wellness* and *well-being* are big buzzwords, and thankfully there are a ton of options in terms of techniques and tools to live well. But so many choices can also be daunting: *Which ones should you choose? When should you integrate them into your life?* It can be confusing. This section will help you identify what techniques and tools to use when, and leaves the door open for you to incorporate the wellness practices you are already using.

Just as we practice yoga and meditation on a regular basis for our health and state of mind, with Slow Beauty you will also have the opportunity to practice a fun, healthy, lifestyle throughout your day. Over time, that lifestyle becomes who you are. *Slow Beauty* will provide you with a host of rituals that can be performed both on a daily and intermittent basis to enhance your life and light you up from the inside. In this section you'll find a huge variety of ways to do this, including hydration, movement, light therapy (in other words, aligning ourself with our built-in circadian rhythm), and ideas for group gatherings. This diverse menu allows you to go however wide and deep you choose to, and to adjust that scope as you evolve and the various seasons of life come and go.

The ultimate goal with all of this is to better attune yourself with your mind, body, and energy levels on both a day-to-day and a seasonal basis, and to help you live your life in an intentional way. As I've seen in my own Slow Beauty practice and in my work with others, once you discover how alive and refreshed you feel from incorporating these rituals and how permissive and accepting you feel when you understand your natural cycles of downtime, you will fall into an easy routine of awareness and self-care that will leave you joyful, enlivened, and brimming with self-acceptance. With these practices incorporated into our daily life, we improve with time, rather than fading away. The passage of time becomes something to celebrate rather than to fear. This, my friends, is true freedom.

RECIPES

Whether we're ingesting them or applying them, Mother Nature has armed us with all of the ingredients we need to keep our body running like a well-oiled machine. Here, you will learn how to put nature's bounty to good use through recipes for teas, soups, juices, infused waters, and smoothies, which bolster body, mind, and spirit. When we're talking about recipes as they pertain to Slow Beauty, though, it includes more than just what we put into our mouth. It also involves being dedicated to ensuring that we put only the best *on* our body as well so as to promote recovery and vitality.

With that in mind, I'll also be sharing a variety of deliciously effective recipes, such as sugar scrubs, body oils, mists, and soaks. I love using homemade beauty products not only because they allow us to control and have a greater awareness of what we're putting on our body, but also because we can cater them to what we need at any given moment in time, whether it's a bit of hydration during the hot summer months or a soothing concoction to counteract the effects of harsher winter conditions. These treatments will be organized by season so that you can better align yourself with the natural rhythms of the world around you.

We'll also cover some more intangible recipes. For example, I will lead you through the process of creating your own mantras for the purposes of self-affirmation, a more optimistic outlook, and manifestation. I will also share a variety of physical movements designed for various seasons. While these will help tone and refine the body, they are all, at heart, meditative in nature and will thus enhance your mental, emotional, and spiritual fitness, as well.

The recipes included in this book will not only leave you looking and feeling great, but they will also help you break down the obstacles in your life. I know—sounds like a big promise, right? Here's why it works: By putting good things on your body and in your body and mind, you will ultimately feel better about yourself and enjoy an improved body image. This will be your greatest protection against the constant barrage of beauty ideals being incessantly hurled at us from every direction. From this wonderful place, you will naturally begin to discover the unique gifts that lie within you, as opposed to wasting your energy striving to become a part of an idealized standard. Obviously, this will leave you feeling great, but it's also an act of altruism because once you've unearthed your gifts, you can contribute them to the world.

MAPPING

Slow Beauty is a philosophy, but how each individual practices it should feel different because *we* are all different and unique. Beauty is a way of life with countless compositions of varying sizes, shapes, forms, and colors. Just as there is not one catchall variety of outer physical beauty, neither is there one for internal beauty. Sure, there are many universal tips and tricks that I can (and will!) offer you, but it's also vital that each of us caters our own Slow Beauty routine to the uniquely beautiful creature we are and to those specific things in life that bring us joy and peace.

With all of this in mind, I am especially excited about the final Mapping section of this book because *this* is really the essence of Slow Beauty and what we're ultimately striving for. It is here that you will really get in touch with your own path—where you are at right now, where you want to go, and how you will get there. For each of us, those answers are beautifully personal. Through a series of written, artistic, and mental exercises, I will offer you an avenue for digging into that deepest part of yourself to find what specific things you need to realize the full strength, energy, and luminous beauty of your inner core.

you write the slow beauty user's manual: practice makes process

The ideas in this book are both additive and subtractive—you can build on what you are already doing *and* you can easily drop anything you find in here that simply isn't resonating with you. It is through this process of developing your own Slow Beauty practice that you will have the opportunity to get to know yourself better; to get in touch with your inner wisdom; and to shut out all of the outside noise and influences to find that core of what makes you joyful.

Most important, I encourage you to *engage* with this book. Make it your own! Have a pen by you at all times so that you can circle words that call out to you, make notes, or doodle. Underline, draw in it, dog-ear it, highlight, write in the margins, react, glue things to the pages, add pages— anything goes. This is *your* book, and your book should have your process all over it. The idea is to transform it into something that is meaningful to you. It's meant to be referenced again and again, carried around as a companion, and the rituals and recipes tried and tweaked to suit your personal style and taste.

What's more is that, although you are creating your own program, you don't have to go it alone! Of course you may do this as a solitary practice if you wish, but Slow Beauty is also set up in such a way that you can build a community around it to support your process, and, through this, you can also support others. (In fact, on page 75 I will show you how to form a group to develop your Slow Beauty practice.) What I want to emphasize is that this book is simultaneously very personal and very communal. But, most of all, it's whatever works for you. This is in no way a rigid, prescriptive, follow-the-rules-or-else tome. It's a joyful, living, breathing, and liberating practice; not something to be perfected, but something that is always in process, just like the changing, evolving, human being you are.

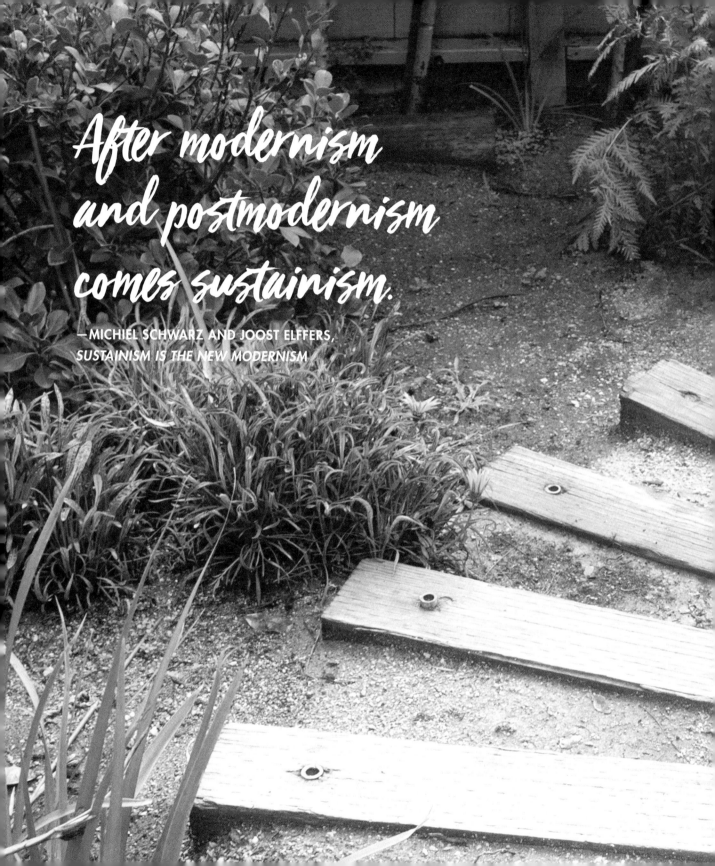

After modernism
and postmodernism
comes sustainism.

—MICHIEL SCHWARZ AND JOOST ELFFERS,
SUSTAINISM IS THE NEW MODERNISM

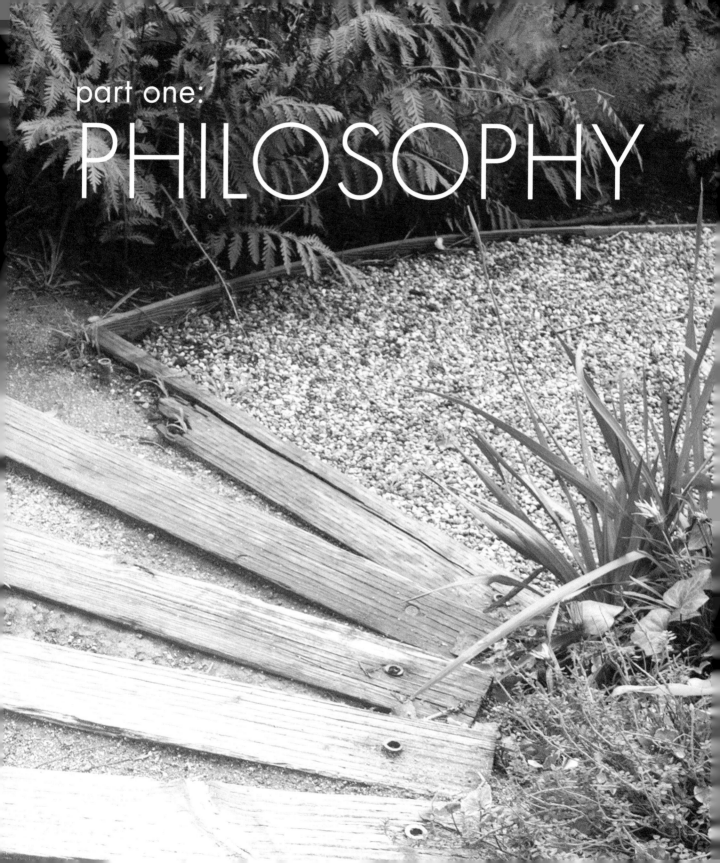

part one:
PHILOSOPHY

my satori moment

Eight years ago, my son's class pet, Torti, came to stay at our house for a couple of weeks. At that point in time I, like so many others, was just being immersed in the world of smartphones and social media, and the constant connection that comes with that. It just felt like everything was moving so fast and going nonstop. And then there was Torti. Mesmerized, I would lose time watching that tortoise move about with his slow, deliberate walk. It seemed almost as though he was in a constant state of meditation. He existed fully within each moment and was happy simply to walk, one intentional step at a time. It was beautiful to witness. In Native American medicine, tortoises appropriately represent mindfulness and patience. Torti certainly reminded me of how important those two things are.

I had a revelation during the course of those two weeks with Torti, or what is known as a satori moment in the Zen tradition. As I watched this ancient creature move slowly but purposefully about, I realized that this was exactly what I'd been practicing for my entire life. And, in that moment of solidarity with Torti, I finally had a name for what I'd been doing all along and understood how to bring it into the world: Slow Beauty.

Slow Beauty provides practitioners with a framework for living their life through its rituals and practices. We start slowly, and then build from there. Slow Beauty involves a philosophy and a series of rituals and recipes that guide you through the process of treating yourself well and living your life in such a way that you will flip on that inner light switch. (Actually, I want you to more specifically think of a dimmer switch—a light that has lots of other settings besides just On and Off.) This practice will help you find peace, happiness, contentment, and self-love in the process; nourish your body, mind, and soul; and, as a result, you will look more beautiful and feel more ageless than ever before. Best of all, Slow Beauty allows you to "map" your own well-being regimen, ensuring that your journey is personalized and uniquely caters to you.

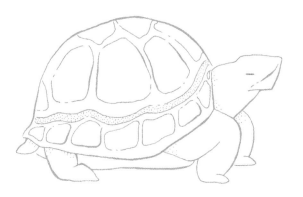

the seeds of slow beauty

I had the good fortune of growing up with a mom who marched to the beat of her own drummer. I grew up in the 1970s and '80s, the height of unnatural shades of makeup, and an abundance of hairspray. As a testament to the era, I remember one particular instance when I put every single color of eye shadow on my eyes at the same time. We had the latest issues of *Vogue* and *Harper's Bazaar* in the house at all times. But, amid this, my mom engrained in me lessons about more natural modes of health and wellness. This included beauty, but also extended to how we lived in general. My mom was into alternative therapies, such as iridology (studying the eye to determine a patient's systemic health) and reflexology. She had dairy delivered to our house in glass containers because she was suspicious of plastic. She taught me how to read the ingredient labels on beauty products, showing me both what to look for and what to avoid. The lifestyle my mom promoted in our house was in huge contrast to the chemical warfare that was being quietly waged around us. In fact, the book *Silent Spring*—an early environmental book that discusses the detrimental effects of pesticides and the chemical industry in general—mentions the pesticide spraying in the Michigan suburb where I grew up. Everyone thought my mom was eccentric at the time, but it turned out she was just several steps ahead of the world at large.

Don't get me wrong. My mom loved all things beauty and fashion—it's just that she was conscious about her choices. From a young age, my mom took me with her to the spa, but she stressed its benefits as a tool for health and wellness, rather than for enhancing outer beauty. Her entire ethos was "health is wealth." "After all," she would say, "If we don't have our health, what do we have?"

When the time came for me to go out into the world on my own, I was armed with this sense of health and wellness my mom had instilled in me. When I went to college, I sought out yoga, which, at the time, was far from a mainstream practice. In fact, I had to go off campus to take classes with a lovely group of senior citizens who welcomed me with open arms. After college, I moved to Los Angeles and took up Transcendental Meditation. I found an Ayurvedic doctor at—of all places—a mall in Topanga Canyon. I was constantly seeking new modalities that made me feel more alive and invigorated, and that provided me with better, natural ways of taking care of myself. People often comment about how young I look. I attribute all of this to the fact that it's simply engrained in me to take good care of myself, working primarily on the inside, and supporting this with holistic external self-care practices. Even after an entire lifetime of living like this, I continue to see myself evolving and growing. So, while some people dread the passage of time, I embrace it. The more time passes, the more deeply I delve into myself. And the more I connect with me, the more beautiful and at peace with myself I feel. This is true for all of us.

flipping the switch on

Turning on your inner light (or *enlightenment*) is just one term for the effect Slow Beauty will have on you. You might also view it through the lens of growing younger, raising your consciousness, vibrating at a higher energy level, or existing in a state of bliss. All of these feelings are a result of a phenomenon psychologist Abraham Maslow termed *self-actualization*. You've probably heard of self-actualization before. It's one of those buzzwordy phrases that can be a bit difficult to nail down.

Well, guess what? Maslow also identified some of the signs that self-actualization *has* happened or is in the process of happening. As you move through the Slow Beauty program, we'll check in to note if you are experiencing any of these symptoms of self-actualization or awakening—both of which are key steps along the path to enlightenment. Let's start with where you're at today to get a baseline. Under each of these markers of self-actualization, determine where you are on a scale of 1 to 10, with 10 being the most proficient. But, first, take a deep breath. This is not a test and there are no right or wrong answers. As you move through *Slow Beauty* you will be amazed to flip back to this and see what has changed and shifted. And, indeed, things *will* change and shift!

Efficient perception of reality: Are you right here, right now? Or are you living in the past or dreaming of the future?

Acceptance of self, others, and nature: Do you truly understand that there is no such thing as failure? As long as we learn from our mistakes, there are only lessons learned.

Spontaneity: Do you know who you are and are you able to stay focused on what you need? It is through this that you will be able to take immediate action in ways that propel you toward the realization of your goals.

Problem-centering (as opposed to ego-centering): Are you able to focus on the issue at hand at any given moment? Can you refrain from complaining or internalizing situations?

Detachment and the desire for privacy: Do you regularly and consistently create time for solitude to check in with yourself and to recharge your battery?

Autonomy and resistance to enculturation: Do you challenge the norm? Don't sign on to something just because others have.

Continued freshness of appreciation and richness of emotional reactions and experiences: Are you able to revel in your sensory experiences for a greater appreciation of your environment and of those around you?

Deep interpersonal relationships: Do you experience relationships that are based on psychological trust and elevated communication? How we engage in dialogue with others is a powerful reminder that we are creating our world with our speech and thoughts.

Democratic character structure: Are you able to address and treat the collective mind, body, and spirit? It is in doing this that we experience what it means to be truly beautiful.

Greatly increased creativity: Are you able to clear any energy that is weighing you down? This opens the channels for self-expression.

Certain changes in your value system: Are you working toward more mindful living? Toward a way of life in which you know what you think and feel and are able to express your needs clearly, concisely, and confidently?

As Walter Truett Anderson says in his book *The Next Enlightenment*, enlightenment is already here, all around us. The problem is that there are obstacles and barriers that keep us from *waking up* to this enlightenment. If you are experiencing this in your own life, there are some exercises in the Rituals section of this book (beginning on page 43) that will help you identify and break down the barriers that are keeping you from experiencing life as a blessing.

beauty with substance— it's an inside job

Enlightenment is a lofty goal. I'm not suggesting that we all strive to walk around like Buddha every day of our life. Beauty is not—and I repeat, *not*—a pursuit of perfectionism. Anyway, we are already perfect! Slow Beauty isn't about beauty as we've always known it—and it's certainly not about the Photoshopped perfection that pervades our culture today.

Slow Beauty is a complete revolution to our thinking about and relationship with beauty. Through this practice, we are redefining beauty together, not as media and mainstream advertising tell us it should be. This isn't to deny that there's an external element to beauty, either. Of course there is! Who doesn't love to acknowledge and admire a beautiful face, body, or work of art? Or the awesomeness of a breathtaking display of nature? For some reason, though, we have defined and related to beauty as something that lives only on the surface. And when something doesn't fit the cultural standard, we ostracize and marginalize it.

The Japanese have philosophies around this, such as *wabi sabi*, which is all about finding beauty in imperfection and transience, feeling a profound connection to the earth, and honoring authenticity above all else. It requires the courage to accept things as they are and that we slow down to appreciate things as they are. There's another Japanese concept called *kintsigu*. Kintsigu is about recognizing, accepting, and drawing near to you the beauty of what is broken. Instead of discarding what is broken, kintsigu asks us to slow down and take the time to repair the object with "golden thread." We can learn a lot about beauty from both wabi sabi and kintsigu. Both speak to bringing near and radically accepting and being inclusive of those parts of ourself that we have marginalized, ostracized, or banished to the wastelands. Both philosophies speak to radical self-compassion, deep caring, deep knowing, and extreme kindness. Also, I just love the idea of fixing something with golden thread. Gold has so many beautiful connotations, including light, strength, and treasure. Particularly with kintsigu, broken objects are elevated by the use of gold to bind them together, resulting in more beauty than the object could have possessed before the break. It is a reminder that it is the breaks, cracks, holes, and chips that make us unique and truly beautiful. It calls to mind a Hasidic saying in the Jewish tradition: "There is nothing more whole than a broken heart." Those of us existing in the world today can learn a lot from these centuries-old ideas about finding beauty in so-called imperfections.

Here in Western culture, we haven't delved below the epidermis; we haven't peeked inside, behind the veil. And that's why there is the breakdown, the decay of the integrated self; because the foundation, the underneath, the *depth* hasn't been addressed, cultivated, loved, cared for, acknowledged, understood, or seen in the way it needs to be seen. True beauty runs deep and it runs clean. The skin is our largest organ, yes; but our mind is our processor, and our spirit communicates with the invisible. So, how we nourish our mind, body, and spirit needs to be intentional and mindful. Step by step, we need to infuse these three overlapping and interconnected circles with meaningful, intentional, nourishing, profound rituals and recipes to go deeper and achieve real, high-functioning, optimal, sustainable beauty. It's an inside job. Inner beauty—beauty from the inside out—it's all within. We've all heard the terms, but we have trouble defining what they actually mean. Slow Beauty will help you create your own definition of beauty.

slow = sustainable

Just a few pages into this book and already, we keep bumping into this idea of sustainability. How does it tie into beauty? Much like the concept of sustainability has swept through the culinary and environmental sectors of our culture, it is the next logical movement in the beauty world as well. This philosophy of sustainability is based on a long-term lifestyle approach to beauty, as opposed to quick fixes and results that are solely external. Similar to how the world is turning away from pumping up our food with chemicals to make it grow faster and to make it appear "healthier" and more vibrant (while simultaneously stripping it of its true character and damaging its composition), we must also do the same for our own selves. What we are essentially accomplishing through the practice of Slow Beauty is tapping into the wisdom of beauty by creating a *sustainable* program that keeps us true to who we are and how we're made. This is a personal process that cannot be done with a snap of the fingers or with a cut-and-dried 1-2-3 formula.

I'm sure it will come as absolutely no surprise to you that the verdict is in: We are all stressed out. In fact, it's so bad that this word, *stress*, is even a part of the vernacular of children less than ten years old. When I was growing up, stress was an elusive concept, reserved solely for adults. Now everyone is feeling the intensity; stress knows no boundaries and has no minimum age limit. How can we feel truly beautiful on the inside when we're living under these conditions?

In this fast-moving, hyperconnected world, more sustainable ways of living have never been more important in *every* facet of our life. Without it, we are all flirting with burnout as we have never seen before. Slow Beauty is yet another way to incorporate into your life this philosophy of sustainability that goes hand in hand with slowing down. Sustainability is about the long term, the long haul, the long run. It's about endurance and process. It is cyclical, collaborative, interconnected, and holistic. This is precisely why sustainability *must* be at the heart of such a practice as Slow Beauty.

The process we're talking about in these pages supports you in designing a holistic, interconnected ecosystem for optimal mind-, body-, spirit-communication. This goes beyond products. I guarantee you this: No matter how far you extend your search or how much you are willing to pay for it, there isn't a pill or procedure on this earth that can replace sustainable self-care. If you are looking for something fast and temporary, then Slow Beauty isn't for you. (And if you *are* looking for a quick fix, I encourage you to ask yourself why you need instant results. What's the rush?) If, on the other hand, you are seeking something eternal,

infinite, and supportive of a higher consciousness and higher quality of life, then continue. Join us. We need you. The world needs you.

All of this is simply a reminder of those things we already know. We just have to wake up to it, pull the pieces together, and embrace our whole, slow self. Wake up, Sleeping Beauty!

Looking at beauty through this filter of sustainability may sound somewhat revolutionary now, but I firmly believe that soon it will not be "alternative" at all. It will be the new norm. This Slow Beauty movement begins on an individual basis. *You* are necessary because it is one by one that this shift will happen: first, you will do it for yourself and your own well-being; then, you will serve as an example for others. And, finally, the entire world will catch on to this more beautiful, more fulfilling, more joyful way of living.

Slow Beauty is activism for the self. It is a social justice movement for the self. Far too often, we behave as if we are at war with ourself. We focus on "antiaging," we fight against time, we admonish the natural process and beauty of aging, and we terrorize ourself with our inner language about this process. Our internal dialogue is mean, harsh, overly critical, and negative. It overflows into how we speak about ourself to others, and how we speak about others, too. We've been estranged from our biggest ally—ourself. Ultimately, Slow Beauty isn't about aging, slow aging, or antiaging. It's about an entirely new idea: holding youth.

the fountain of youth exists within

I like to imagine the positive implications of a world in which we grew young instead of old. How we currently age is tied up in the socialization processes into which we are born. We are assigned phases of life: birth, adolescence, adulthood, old age, and death. Within those phases, we are prescribed to follow certain psychological, emotional, physical, and financial milestones each step of the way. We blindly follow this consumptive path, and if we veer off it or it doesn't work for us, we are ostracized not only by others but, even worse, by ourself. It doesn't *have* to be this way.

Imagine if when we were born people told us stories about how we would grow young instead of "preparing" us for the fact that we would someday grow old, decay (in a prescribed home for the aged), and die (and, with death and dying in our culture comes the connotation of something very far from beauty). It's as if, from the very beginning, life and time are framed as a curse, rather than the blessing they really are. How nonsensical is that?! The trickle-down effects of thinking differently and shifting our focus from growing old to growing young are monumental. If we are able to make this seis-mic shift in perception and relinquish the idea that we are solely chronologically aging, we will also shed all of the biases that come along with our ideas about aging. As things stand now, the aging process has been commoditized. Growing old is the bait, and we have bitten into it hook, line, and sinker. Aging—and our resulting attempts to ward it off with "antiaging" products and procedures—has become a self-fulfilling prophecy of decay, instead of a glorious celebration of the full life we are born to live.

In his book *Growing Young*, anthropologist Ashley Montagu has identified twenty-seven behavioral needs of human beings that, when developed and nurtured throughout an entire lifetime, enable us to "hold youth" rather than growing old. To satisfy these needs, we need to exercise them indefinitely (in other words, they need to be sustainable—there's that word again!). These needs must become something we engender throughout our lifetime, rather than things we only experience as children, then later eschew because they aren't sanctioned "adultlike" behaviors.

Of these twenty-seven needs, Montagu states that the "humanizing need," love, stands at the

center of all others. And *that* is one of the huge keys to this Slow Beauty philosophy we're talking about: exercising the most radical, extreme, deep, profound, compassionate love for ourself. Maybe you weren't loved the way you needed to be loved in childhood, or perhaps you aren't experiencing love the way you need to right this very moment. Here I offer you an intimate, personal practice of self-care that, when put into action, will connect you with and give you a better understanding of the ways in which you need to be loved and—most vital of all—how you need to love yourself. No matter how overwhelming it may seem to even begin to crack that code of what your needs are right now, soon you will understand not only what they are, but also how to satisfy them. Before long, you will reflect this same love that you're giving yourself back into the world and into your relationships. Guess what happens then? That love comes full circle, and is reflected back at you, creating an incredibly gorgeous cycle.

Perhaps you're intrigued—you really, *really* want it—but you're still a bit overwhelmed? Here's some more good news for you: The greatest gift of being human is that we are always *becoming*. So, no matter what age we are chronologically, we still have the opportunity to cultivate within ourself these human needs that Montagu speaks of. And not only that, but we have the opportunity to deeply *experience* them. This is both a very spiritual concept, and the end result of a sequence of biological occurrences. As Montagu himself put it:

Konrad Lorenz, the German ethologist, writing in 1950, maintained that by far the more important features in the investigation of human evolution are not physical but behavioral. He drew heavily on the ideas of the German sociologist Arnold Gehlen, who recognized as early as 1940 that the unique human trait is that of remaining in an unending state of development. The specialty of human beings is non-specialization; humans have remained free to change as change is required by whatever environment they encounter; they are able to develop special traits to meet special needs. Lorenz holds that these traits are behavioral as well as physical. *

Throughout this book we will engage in exercises, rituals, recipes, and thinking that will help us tap into Montagu's twenty-seven basic human needs, many of which we have neglected due to the biases of the environments in which we have been raised or find ourself in now. We will nurture these needs and integrate them into our mind, body, and spirit so that they may support our beautiful becoming.

What better time to start than right now?

*All Montagu quotes in Part One excerpted from *Growing Young* by Ashley Montagu.

montagu's twenty-seven basic human needs

As you review this list of needs, read both the word and its definition out loud. Take your time as you go. Be slow. Notice what each of these needs incites within you, whether it's a physical sensation, a feeling, a memory, or anything else.

Write down your own definition and any other thoughts, ideas, and experiences that come up around that idea. Don't edit. Don't judge. Just let it flow. Another way to work with these needs, reinforce them, and internalize their wisdom is to commit to working with one per week over a twenty-eight-week period (as you'll see, I added one of my own in addition to Montagu's twenty-seven) and to go deep with it. Begin by similarly writing the definition and your thoughts and ideas about it, but then go deeper by practicing the need, talking about it, and maybe even creating a Women's Gathering (see page 75) built around a discussion of and working with this particular need. Get inside that need, and allow it to get inside of you, to become you.

① LOVE

Montagu highlights love as *the* standout essential need that should be central to our life. We need outlets to share and show our love in the ways that we individually know how. We also need to receive love in the form we require. Love, in its truest, most unconditional form, is the best and most powerful variety of medicine. As you read this book and think about love, think about the ways in which you need to express your love, and the ways in which you choose to be loved. "Out of the learning of love grows the love of learning. It is the consistent exercise of the ability to love that humanizes us, that makes us human."

② FRIENDSHIP

Another form of love, friendship is important for the development of "good human relations." Think about the type of friend you are or would like to be and what type of friends you would like to have. List your tribe of friends and think about the ways you nurture those friendships. Friendship is something to be cherished and nourished; we must weave the threads of trust together. Maybe you are someone who is very social and has a lot of friends, or perhaps you only have a few very close friends. Maybe you are your own bestie, or maybe your partner is. Perhaps, as was the case with poets Mary Oliver and Walt Whit-man, nature is your trusted friend. Whatever form friendship takes for you, it's all wonderful.

③ SENSITIVITY

We live in a world where we're often told we're too sensitive, yet sensitivity is key to experiencing the depth of life. This need is being challenged in today's world, where we are so caught up in profits and the bottom line, at the expense of the health and happiness of human beings. We need to go deeper with our experience of self, others, and life. "Sensitivity deepens the experience of what life has to offer and enlarges our apprehension and appreciation of it." Next time someone says, "You are too sensitive," be sure to thank the person, because you are exactly what the world needs right now, at this very moment in time.

④ THINK SOUNDLY

We are moving at such a fast pace that we have forgotten the importance of observation, analysis, and experimental thinking. We are overly focused on instant results, instant answers, and instant responses. How quickly and thoughtlessly do you respond to texts, e-mails, and Instagram comments? It's important to slow down and be self-reflective. We need to set some boundaries to keep the distractions that are preventing us from thinking soundly at bay.

⑤ TO KNOW

To be deeply involved in your passion leads you to knowing. This knowing has profound implications on your mind, body, and spirit. It gives you a foundation upon which to expand your sense of authentic self.

⑥ TO LEARN

Play to learn and orient yourself to always be learning. You can learn something from everyone and every situation, every day. Waking up with the thought "What will I learn today?" will keep you in an ongoing state of mental and consciousness expansion. It is when we have the false belief that we already know everything that we become stagnant. Learning is life. A lifelong love of learning keeps the mind flexible, youthful, and enlightened.

⑦ TO WORK

We learn the most about ourself from the work we do. We should think of our work as a work of art versus just a job or a way of paying our bills. Find the art in your work. And if you do not find it, then find the work that contains the art for you. Being content in your work lights up your life and illuminates you. Do work that allows you the chance to really get to know yourself and what you are made of.

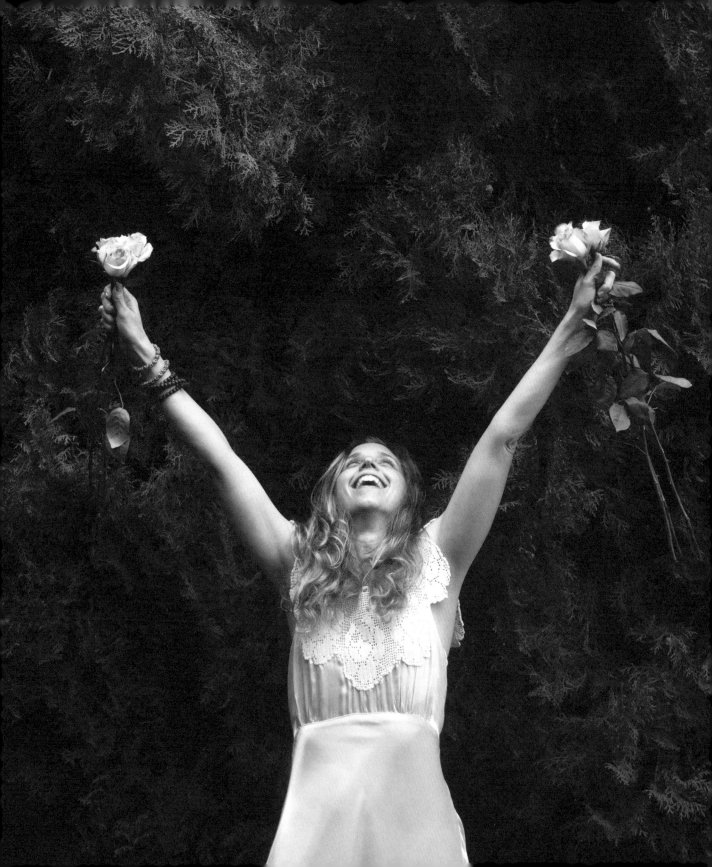

(8) ORGANIZATION

We need organization for clarity of mind, focus, and intention. An organized mind is an enlightened mind. When our mind becomes cluttered with distractions and overburdened by too many choices, it's a signal that it is time to slow down and shrug off some of our mental clutter.

(9) CURIOSITY

This need speaks to the vigor of the mind, and its unquenchable need to explore. Curiosity is something to be encouraged and celebrated. Ask questions, probe, turn over stones, look under rocks. Be relentlessly inquisitive.

(10) WONDER

A sense of wonder deeply corresponds with life itself. It is an interest, an awe that contains the essence of excitement and possibilities. Wonder is a need that holds expectation, and "participation in the known and unknown." Wonder opens the door to the mysteries of life, to the invisible, eternal, infinite inner workings of life.

(11) PLAYFULNESS

Playfulness is where joy resides. Play leads to innovation, it propels us beyond our habits and our comfort zones. There is an element of surprise, spontaneity, and imagination in play. This concept of the "inner child" is not a cliché, but a real, valuable need to be emotionally, mentally, and physically healthy. Play with your thoughts, your ideas, your words, your exchanges with others, and your movements. Approach life through a lens of playfulness. Play in your friendships and with your loves. Be playful with yourself. Play to stay young for eternity. Play to keep life fresh and alive.

(12) CREATIVITY

Creativity is why we need to express ourself. When we are satisfying this need, we are healthy. When we are creative and encouraged to create, we are in a process of becoming—we are fluid, in movement, engaged, and enriched. When we create, we embrace change. We flow with the current of life instead of flailing against it.

(13) OPEN-MINDEDNESS

We need this to maintain a healthy relationship with all of humanity. When we are open-minded, we become free from prejudice and rigidness, and we are more respectful to the ideas and concerns of others. With an open mind, we are able to connect to our self and others in much deeper and more meaningful ways.

(14) FLEXIBILITY

A flexible mind is a mind that extends itself in all directions. It is a mind always in pursuit of growth. It grows through deep listening and consideration of opinions. When new evidence presents itself, the mind flexes to adapt, rethink, and reconsider. It is a mind that is both respectful of tradition and open to the new. Flexibility requires us to challenge all prejudices, and pursue beauty and truth in the name of self and life itself.

15 EXPERIMENTAL-MINDEDNESS

What type of thinker are you? When you think experimentally, you become an observer, setting up hypotheses and then testing them to see whether they are true. When you are an observer, your range of life experience is larger—it has more longitude and latitude, more texture, and more sensuality.

16 EXPLORATIVENESS

Being an explorer of life is being alive. When we explore we are engaged, we care, we are aware, we are deeply interested, and we are intrigued. Exploration has no boundaries; we can explore nature, culture, books, architecture, all expressions of art, and so much more.

17 RESILIENCE

How long does it take you to bounce back from a challenge or something that has rattled you? This time frame will give you an idea of how resilient you are. Resilience encourages us to make that "bounce back time" as short as possible. We want to process those stresses that show up in our daily life quickly so we have more freedom to enjoy the fullness of life.

18 ENTHUSIASM

This is joie de vivre, literally "joy of life." Enthusiasm is excitement and exciting. It is infectious. It gets things done, motivates others to get things done, uplifts, and energizes. Enthusiasm is real, authentic, and earnest.

19 SENSE OF HUMOR

Find ways to laugh at yourself. A sense of humor loosens and frees us from the harsh realities of suffering and banality. It adds texture, color, shape, and taste to what is otherwise boring and stagnant. A sense of humor lightens the load and colors what is otherwise dull and gray. Humor erupts at the intersection of the unexpected and incompatible.

20 JOYFULNESS

Joy is a quintessential need most connected to the spiritual realm. It is an essence that is fluid, creative, regenerative, and enduring. Joy is vital. Joy is always young and always an access point to growing young. With joy there is no chronological aging, it is boundless, and without boundaries. Joy is pure life.

21 AND 22 LAUGHTER AND TEARS

Laughter is the realest of the real. It is a glorious outburst of authenticity. The smile that accompanies laughter is the personification of friendliness and warmth. Laughter is healing. And so are tears. Tears cleanse, rebalance, recalibrate, restore, soften, and open a hardened heart. Laughter and tears enjoin feelings of goodness, wholeness, and renewal. We rejoice in the freedom to laugh and to weep for our mental, physical, and spiritual health.

(23) OPTIMISM

Eternal optimism is a self-fulfilling prophecy of one success after another. When we are oriented toward an optimistic outlook, anything is possible. Optimism is freedom and goodness not only good for the individual, but also for the group at large.

(24) HONESTY AND TRUST

We need to be honest, trusting, and trusted. Often, we are not honest with ourself or others because we are fearful. We need to move beyond these fears to honest expressions of what our needs are, and trust ourself to express those needs. When we build a foundation of trusting ourself by expressing our needs and leaving situations that do not support those needs, it becomes easier to trust others and the world at large.

(25) COMPASSIONATE INTELLIGENCE

We need to care, nurture, nourish, support, and sustain others through this combination of strength and loving kindness. Compassionate intelligence sees potential and helps people rise up. When it sees weakness it does not trample, it reaches out a hand and lifts up. There is no hate, only empathy. There is no fear, only fearlessness to recognize that what we see in others is a part of us too, no matter what. This need reaches across lines, boundaries, fences, and borders. It says, "I understand you," "I am here for you," and "I hear you." It never makes fun, destroys, or knocks down. It smiles, builds up, and puts back together.

(26) DANCE

To just let go and dance is the most amazing feeling. To dance is to be in tune, it is to speak the language of the body, the language of the eternal. When we try the different dances of various world cultures, we better understand who they are because it is in the subtlety and nuances of the movement where their truth lives. There is also a door to freedom in dance, an opportunity to completely relinquish control, fear, rigidness, judgment, and prejudice. Dance loosens all of that and sets us free. When we give ourself permission to really dance, we are dancing with the cosmos, with eternity, with the infinite, with the source. Dance is therapy, renewal, and replenishment. "There is a release and a replenishment of psychic energy that leaves one with an oceanic feeling of freedom from which all constraint has fallen away, in which the free play of the emotions in disciplined response to music has its way. One is infused with lyrical joy."

(27) **SONG**

Singing is the only true way to understand the power of our voice. When we sing, *really sing*, we know our range. When we know this it comes with us wherever we are, allowing us to express clearly what our needs are and what needs to be expressed through us and by us. We need to sing and to hear our voice. We need to know our voice and to love our voice.

And a twenty-eighth need that I can't help but add…

(28) **UNDERSTANDING**

To understand is wisdom actualized. It is the illumination of wisdom.

you are the love story

Let's linger on love for a little bit. After all, what's really more important than that? But let's also talk about love in a different way than we usually do. Consider this: *Each of us is our own love story.*

As a society, we put so much emphasis on the external, at the expense of our own individuation and integration. We've already discussed how we do this when we talk about beauty, but we also do it when we talk about love. So, I implore you to do this one thing: Love yourself. That's it. The elusive beauty secret you've been looking for is that simple. Love yourself, and love all of yourself—*especially* your vulnerabilities and those parts of yourself that are so easy to write off or label as "ugly." Love those areas that are tender or make you feel unsure, insecure, ashamed, or guilty. Love

those parts of yourself that you have ousted to the margins or obscured in the shadows. Make your love for *you* flow freely, openly, without judgment or restrictions, conditions, or constraints, to all parts of yourself, east and west, north and south, along all latitudes and longitudes. Let the love flow freely through the channels of all of the rivers of yourself— through the tributaries, over the mountain ranges, until they deposit into the deltas.

Slow down to silence the chatter, deter the distractions, and make your way back home. To your real home—to yourself. You can think of this as a form of self-initiation. In the Jewish tradition, it's known as *teshuva*, or a return to self, and is addressed each year during the high holy days. In Jungian terms, it's known as individuation, an integration of the anima and animus. In the Chinese philosophy of Taoism, it's the symbiotic and balanced relationship of the yin and the yang. If we want to have the *full* experience of our life destiny versus the prescribed experience—and, really, who wants that?—then it is a journey that is a bit mysterious and unknown. It's a journey that we must take alone, albeit with some guidance, love, and support. It is a journey inward that is marked by dedication, discipline, and joy. It's about self-politicking and being the agent of our own self-transformation. It's self-care as social justice. You are going to become an activist to support yourself in finding and using your voice in the way that will allow you to create the life you want to live, at the pace that supports your sustained well-being.

Whether we recognize it or not, each and every one of us is our very own love story. Regardless of the status of your love life at this particular moment in time, *you* are the one you've been waiting for. You can stop looking outside of yourself for your better half. That better half is already inside of you. You only need to seek it out and to be tenacious in that quest. When you make yourself whole, that's when you will bloom. But first you have to do the work—it takes practice, and it's slow. Precisely *because* this process takes time and discipline and commitment, its results will last for a lifetime. Don't you think it's about time you came home to yourself?

Self-love is not just any old love story, it's *the greatest* love story of all time. Self-love is about communing with yourself to create authentic community. It isn't about being controlled by something outside of yourself that you perceive as being greater than you. It is about your energy levels and understanding how to work with your energy so that you can function at an optimal level. It's about connecting with the higher, elevated, enlightened self that functions above and outside the buzz of all the noise of the world. It is about bearing witness to who you are and who others are instead of being caught up or pulled down into the frenzy or the drama or the chaos. It's about choosing the middle way rather than being pulled in extreme directions. It's about getting back to basics. Health, wellness, well-being, and beauty are accessible to everyone, regardless of age or socioeconomic status. It is our birthright. Nature isn't trendy, and neither is our nature. Kale is still kale even when it's being "replaced" by mushrooms as the new hot ingredient. Regardless of whether or not kale is out of fashion, it still remains one of the most nutrient-dense vegetables and benefits our bones, hair, and skin. Likewise, we are still who we are even when our energy is low, when we feel depressed, irritable, malnourished, and weak. Even with all of this, there is still a strong, joyful, self within who is full of vitality. We are still deserving of our own love.

To uncover your optimal self, you just need to adjust some things, remove others, and add a dash of this and that. With a regular Slow Beauty practice, you can identify potential weaknesses and focus your attention on them to strengthen them before a potential fall. In this way, Slow Beauty is a prevention practice.

A NEW KIND OF LOVE STORY

Speaking of love, maybe it's time we look at these love stories that have been engrained in us since we were little girls from a new perspective. Like many stories we've been told over the centuries, "Cinderella" serves and perpetuates a narrow sense of self and keeps us stuck in outdated gender roles. It teaches women that we are meant to be gorgeously passive as we wait for our hero to save us with kisses and to give us our perfect ending. Instead, we should be taught to be our own savior, and the heroine of our own story.

That's why I love another, more authentic and more empowering, version of this story—the story of a girl named Vasalisa, which means "queen" (very different from the translation of Cinderella's name, which is "ashes").

In *Women Who Run with the Wolves*, author Clarissa Pinkola Estés highlights intuition as the main theme of Vasalisa's story. The only way to connect with our intuition, she argues, is to listen to its still, small voice. To acknowledge it, to nourish it, and to follow it.

Vasalisa the Wise has a similar structure as "Cinderella"—up to a point. Just as does Cinderella's, Vasalisa's mother dies when she is quite young. Prior to her death, Vasalisa's mother gives her a doll and instructs Vasalisa to always keep it in her pocket. This doll is her mother's way of initiating Vasalisa into the rites of intuition. Following her mother's death, Vasalisa's father soon remarries a woman who has two daughters. The mother and daughters are mean to Vasalisa. They are jealous, envious, and exclusionary.

Rather than prepping for a glamorous ball and catching the attention of a prince, the stepmother and stepsisters plot to put out all of the fires in the fireplaces throughout their home, and then send Vasalisa out into the forest to request fire from the frightening old hag Baba Yaga. As Vasalisa makes her way through the forest, the doll in her pocket jumps up and down to direct Vasalisa toward Baba Yaga's hut. Once she arrives, the ugly and scary Baba Yaga tells Vasalisa she will only give her the fire after she has passed a series of tests. And if Vasalisa *doesn't* pass these tests, Baba Yaga will eat her.

With no fairy godmother in sight, Vasalisa passes each test with the aid of her intuition. Through the process, she learns her intuition will direct her well and keep her safe. Which, indeed, it does. At last, Vasalisa passes Baba Yaga's final test. Although Baba Yaga would love to eat the girl, she is a just witch and has no choice but to give her the fire for which she came. She puts it in a skull on a stick and Vasalisa, again with the guidance of her intuition, makes her way back to reignite the fireplaces at her stepmother's home. As she approaches the house with the flaming skull, Vasalisa's stepmother and stepsisters run out to greet her, surprised and elated. They are grateful Vasalisa has returned because they were unable to get the fireplaces going again while she was away, and they thought for sure that Baba Yaga had eaten Vasalisa as they had originally hoped. When the skull came into the view of the stepmother and stepsisters, it burned them all to a pile of little ashes.

So, there you have it! Vasalisa, enmeshed by jealousy, envy, and exclusion, is cast away deep into the forest to meet her demise. Instead, she integrates with wild nature and prevails because she listens to her intuition, a blessing from her beloved mother, and passes a series of tests that teach her discernment. Vasalisa returns as a wiser version of herself and with her own well-deserved and powerful light, which sheds light on what does not serve or support her and burns it all away.

Vasalisa shows us how to go out into the deep, dark wilderness within and find and retrieve the light. The story shows us how to find what we need to be our own savior. This story is a perfect example of radical self-love and the rewards of listening to the intuition, going it alone, facing our fears, and returning triumphant.

self-love and narcissism are not the same

The ideas of self-love and self-care are intricately connected. Self-care is taking the time, making the space, and cultivating a wonderful world for you. How many other people in your life do you do this for? And why do you do it? Is it because you love them? Try directing some of this love back to yourself. Use it to fuel that advocacy, to fuel the self-care that is so critical to a Slow Beauty practice—and, moreover, that is critical to your best life, to the life you deserve.

The topic of love has been discussed and dissected since time immemorial. There are songs about love, dances about love, poetry about love, plays about love, movies about love, and television shows about love. In Plato's *Symposium*, philosophers have an in-depth debate about the essence of love, arguing multiple viewpoints. In *The Art of Loving*, social psychologist Erich Fromm discusses the many aspects of love, including everything from the love of God to erotic love to self-love. There are so many facets of love, so many ways to love and be loved, so many different forms and expressions of love—we love our lovers, our friends, our parents, and our children, each in unique ways.

But there's one type of love that we're not so enamored with. And that is self-love. As a society, we have been taught that self-love is a neurosis. That neurosis has a name: narcissism or vanity. Perhaps you've heard the Greek myth about Narcissus, the selfish young man who felt nothing but disdain for everyone who loved him and was banished by the gods to roam the forest in hopes that he would learn from his mistakes.

The soul needs love as urgently as the body needs air. In the warmth of love, the soul can be itself.

—JOHN O'DONOHUE, *ANAM CARA*

Instead, Narcissus became so mesmerized by his own reflection in the pond that he forgot to drink the water and ended up dying of thirst. The term *narcissism* was coined at the turn of the nineteenth century by Havelock Ellis and Paul Näcke and deemed a disorder of "excessive selfishness," stemming from "self-love." In the twentieth century, psychologist Otto Rank solidified narcissism as an unhealthy distortion of self-admiration and vanity. Later, Sigmund Freud, among others, built upon Rank's thesis and this idea of narcissism became engrained in our psyche.

Today, this invention that was inspired by a Greek fable serves as the undertone in many of our personal mythologies. Our dread of narcissism has perverted our experience of self-love, which *should* be a means of wholesomeness, wholeness, and holiness. We aren't taught to love ourself because self-love has been appropriated. Of course there are personality types who truly are narcissistic, but the vast majority of us are not.

We are in awe of great, fabled love affairs; we admire them and yearn for that type of connection for our own. That kind of love that is larger than life, whether it's Cinderella or Romeo and Juliet. The problem with this fixation is that it draws our attention to the external rather than encouraging us to look inward. Ideally we want to first generate love internally—we want to love ourself before looking outward. Of course, love doesn't always happen in that order, and that's okay because self-love is *always* an option. We just need to make the decision to go for it. This self-love, this radical self-care, requires you to be your own most intimate friend, to start being your own soul friend.

We have never been educated about how to love ourself. In fact, most of us have been unconsciously trained to do the opposite. I suppose if we aren't directed to love ourself, if this isn't upheld as a cultural or societal value or a virtue, and if we aren't shown ways in which to achieve self-love, then we will inevitably turn outward to seek external objects to satisfy this very natural, human longing—this human *need*.

That seeking propels us toward the endless consumption of things that never quite satisfy our longings. I'm happy to say that this is changing. People are waking up. Our collective consciousness is evolving, as we begin to consume more mindfully and recognize the importance of meaningful experiences, both personal and communal. We have the opportunity to learn together and teach one another the value of loving our own self. This will, in turn, help us develop a greater capacity to connect with and love others. Our existential feelings of separateness will become less apparent as we return first to ourself and, from there, make our way back to others, with whom we can share the treasures we've discovered within. Love is the beauty. Beauty is the love.

YOU'RE RUNNING FOR OFFICE!

Being an advocate for yourself and loving yourself includes and is influenced both by how you speak to yourself and by how you speak about yourself to others.

Pretend you're running for the president of your own internal democracy. What is your slogan? Jot down a few ideas, right here, right now. Canvas for yourself. Be an advocate for yourself.

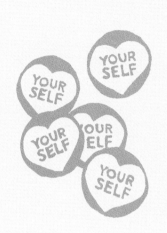

the sign of compromise

Of course, there are times in life when we should compromise; however, there is a balance to this. Compromising too much and too frequently is one of the most insidious enemies of self-love and, by extension, self-care.

I once had a dream where I was walking over some hills. In the midst of that walk I came across a rather large wood sign with the word COMPROMISE clearly etched upon it. Not surprisingly, that sign was relevant to my life at that particular moment, as I'm sure it would be to most people's life at some time or another.

Inevitably, we all make some compromises throughout our lifetime. And to be sure, there are good types of compromises, the ones in which we achieve a mutually agreed upon consensus. And then there is another type of compromise, whereby we settle for things that are below or not aligned with our value system. There are myriad reasons why we may make these types of compromises. At a certain point, though, we need to identify why we are continuing to make them at our own expense. And it doesn't stop with identifying them. From there, we need to *change* our behaviors so that we are stronger when faced with the situations that may lead us to compromise. So that we, again, advocate for ourself in these scenarios.

This way to break this pattern is simple: The next time you find yourself in such a situation, *don't* compromise. Instead, slow down and connect with your inner pace so that you have the time to reflect and feel, to know what is right for you. When you live in this state, you will be able to identify what you need and to give yourself what you love—that self-care and self-love that will break outdated patterns and behaviors, so that, rather than neglecting ourself, we are on the way to becoming our best selves.

healthy, healthier, healthiest

Why is this idea of our own inner pace a cornerstone of the Slow Beauty philosophy and so important to self-love and self-care?

Healthy is beautiful. If we're going to be aspirational here—or, rather, *since* we're going to be aspirational, *healthiest* is our ultimate goal. But getting to that healthiest, most beautiful version of ourself doesn't happen overnight. We want to start by aiming for healthy and build on that. Have patience. This is, after all, a slow-and-steady-wins-the-race philosophy. Be the tortoise, not the hare. Channel Torti.

Slow Beauty is a way of reframing our ideas and ideals about beauty, and expanding our definition of beauty to include health and wellness side by side with the development and design of our inner life. It is about innovating our approach to beauty in such a way that we leave behind the concept of beauty as we've known and experienced it. It's about abandoning altogether our ideas that have us chasing perfectionism and fighting the aging process.

In my mind, the biggest component of any beauty program should be wellness and self-care. Slow Beauty will take you there. It will take you on an interactive wellness and self-care journey that will bring you to a place of optimal health, both inside and out. You will feel the best you've ever felt in your life. And the best part is that you will *continue* to feel good because you are going to personalize your program so that it continues to support and sustain you for the long haul, infinitely, even as you grow and transform and ebb and flow through life.

change is the only stable state in our life

(or: when chaos is a good thing)

It might seem a little bit like I'm talking at cross-purposes here, telling you that you're perfect just the way you are (which is true), and also encouraging you to change.

Here's the thing, though: We live in a world that is inherently changeable. The world around us is always changing and we're always changing, for better or for worse. The point here is to direct that change toward the better in whatever ways are within our control. And, to be sure, not everything is within our control.

Slow Beauty is about two types of change. First, it is about the changing world around us—the type of change that is often beyond our control. It is also about internal change—the "be the change" type that the Dalai Lama so aptly expressed. We need to understand and recognize the sometimes chaotic world around us so that we don't get caught up in the frenzy, lest it swallow us whole. We also want to give ourself the space and the opportunity to change aspects of our life—the things that we do and the habits we've fallen into—to improve how we feel about both ourself and the world around us.

This movement toward change is nothing new. It's just the prescribed manner in which we go about achieving change that shifts from one era to the next. Over the decades the trend of the moment has run the gamut from psychoanalysis to cognitive therapy to "love-ins" to self-help to the pursuit of happiness; from aerobics to Tae Bo to Buns of Steel. The list is exhaustive. Today, we talk about finding change through wellness and well-being. Along the way, certain prominent figures and stories rise to the top, depending on the zeitgeist and what we, as a culture, need to be reflected back to us.

What does this have to do with beauty? Everything. We are always seeking beauty. Human beings are visually oriented beings. We strive for beauty, and we are always in the midst of a discussion about beauty, implicitly or explicitly, whether we realize it or not. We're constantly defining, refining, and redefining standards of beauty based on the social, cultural, and psychological state of the times. *Beautiful* in its most base, common, and banal definition is a transient concept. What was considered beautiful in 1977 is likely not held in the same regard today. In other words, when we chase this sort of culturally defined beauty, we're chasing something that can't really ever be caught. It will always be shifting under our feet and we will constantly be trying to chase it back down. All of this only has to do with physical beauty, though. Slow Beauty, of course, involves the physical because we will always be visual creatures. But it's so much more than that. Slow Beauty is a multisensory experience, and, within that, the visual is only a part of the greater whole.

Time is a funny thing. Einstein (and many other scientists, for that matter) tell us that time doesn't even really exist, that it's nothing more than a human construct. According to this theory, we, as humans, have just collectively applied some labels that represent time as a coping mechanism for what is otherwise a completely chaotic state of countless moving parts. And—here's the kicker—we are just another one of those parts. So, we have the past, present, and future, and we attach meaning and emotions to these timescapes that both hinder and help us. In a sense, time is a line or a thread we can travel along to gain perspective and lessons. It is common for us to reflect on the past, and even to get stuck in the past or be nostalgic for it. Our relationship with the future, on the other hand, is often fraught with worry and concern and a need to control what is to come. In fact, it's probably not news that many of us struggle to be present in the moment.

I've always been fascinated with the future, to the point where I align with the futurists. I'm fascinated and curious about the great art movements of our history—I'm always searching for cues and clues that will give me insight into what is to come so that I will be better prepared.

Slow Beauty is both what is next and what is already here. This desire for wholeness has always been present in us, it's just that now our attention will be more and more attracted to its qualities. Emotionally, psychologically, and physically, we will yearn for it as technological advances appear to accelerate the world around us. We are seeking tools, resources, and the experiences of time standing still.

joy, oh, joy!

I've saved my favorite element of the Slow Beauty philosophy for last: At the end of the day, what we are really doing throughout the course of fostering our own inner beauty, space, and light, is cultivating joy. We are reworking and upgrading our system to ensure that joy runs deep within us, that joy courses through our veins.

Above all else, finding ways to cultivate the spirit of joy within helps us to maintain balance through the ebbs and flows of life. Real joy is rooted deep within and is a key to a spiritually grounded and sustainable self-care practice. Wear joy. The light of joy imparts an exclusive glow. Bask in its warmth. Joy is radiant. Elevated. Fluid.

But what if you are not feeling joy at this particular moment? What if you look within and it seems like it simply doesn't exist? Trust me, *it does*. Even if right now all you have is the tiniest seed of joy, be tenacious in seeking it out. We are going to take that seed and transform it into a majestic, towering, overflowing oak tree.

For some, that idea might feel oddly scary. Yes, there can be fear in the unknown—even when that unknown is joy itself! Be open to the mystery of how you will get there. To the spontaneity of not knowing what's to come. This is where creativity lives—and creativity is inherently joyful. When we create, we know joy.

And guess what? This personalized emotional, spiritual, and physical practice that you have now officially embarked upon is creative. You will create as you slow down, turn inward, and get in touch with, celebrate, and intensify that part of yourself where joy originates.

Now, let's practice!

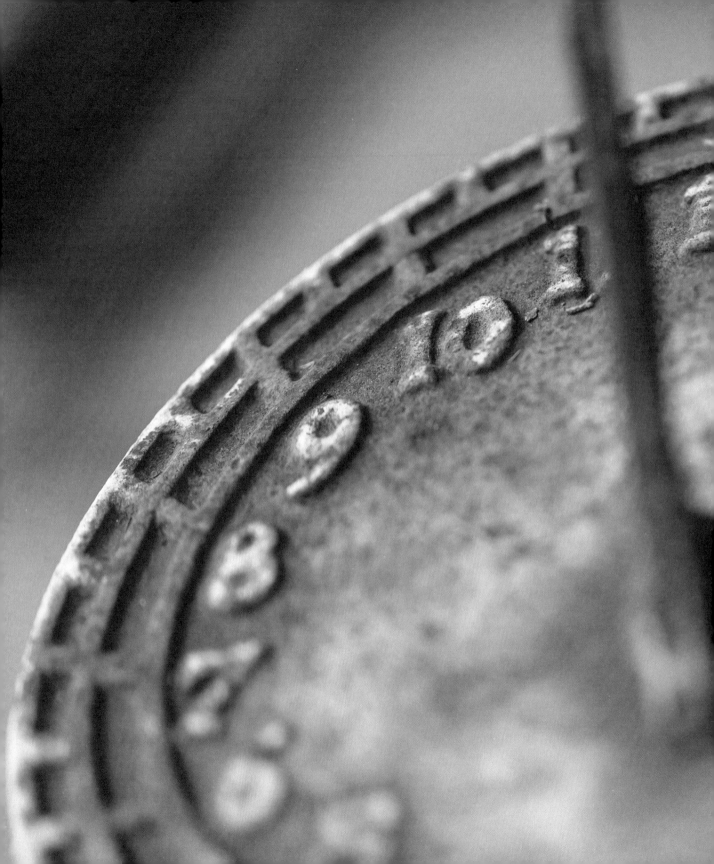

Part Two:
RITUALS

There is a deep beauty within each person. Modern culture is obsessed with cosmetic perfection. Beauty is standardized; it has become another product for sale. In its real sense, beauty is the illumination of your soul.

— JOHN O'DONOHUE, *ANAM CARA*

punctuate your day with rituals

The rituals included in this section provide the framework for incorporating the Slow Beauty philosophy into our life—they are essentially what bring this philosophy close to us as a practice and help us to break down obstacles we've been bumping up against. Through these rituals, we can begin to feel better about ourself and our body, and to gain a sense of agency over our own life. Here I will share some of my favorite rituals, which can be put into practice on a daily, regular, or seasonal basis. You can start as small as you want (perhaps selecting one of these rituals to start) and build from there. The beauty of each of these rituals is that they allow you to begin to lay the groundwork for sustainable self-care. In my experience, once that groundwork is there, it will become easier and more compelling to incorporate more rituals into your life. Not only will these rituals light that inner fire that shines from the inside out, but they will also provide you with some "me" time, allowing you to delve further inside in a way that will ultimately slow you down and bring you in touch with what you need. Some of these rituals are meant to be done in solitude; others are designed to be done with a partner or in a larger group setting.

The uncomfortable thing about rituals is that things will inevitably pop up that are, well, uncomfortable. Undigested material—perhaps an old trauma or unsavory aspects of your upbringing—will rise up to the surface. This is the difficult part of practicing rituals; and yet it is also the pathway to relieve yourself from those aspects of self that no longer serve you. Broken thought records, the ways in which you uncomfortably hold parts of your body, all of these things that cause pain can be ameliorated through the practice of rituals. This section will offer you intentional ways to slow down, to help you unfold, and unfurl aspects of your beauty that have been hidden away from both yourself and from others. Rituals also help you break out of old patterns of doing and being. When we are truly engaged in ritualistic practices, they help us break out of old unhealthy habits and patterns.

So, all of this begs the question: What *are* rituals? They are modes through which we access our self, our inner life, and pathways to making a greater, more intimate connection to our self. We use rituals so that we don't travel too far off of the path away from ourself. Rituals ground us and give shape to our days, our weeks, our months, and our years. They mark a point in time, and bring a sense of meaning and a shape to what otherwise blends in to everything else. Rituals make the ordinary remarkable, and illuminate the banal. Rituals are a pathway to self-transformation. They slow down time. Rituals have a purpose and there are different types to be utilized or set into motion to achieve many different results. Some are used to wake us up out of our routine state, others are meant to move us to a different emotional place, to stimulate our senses, and to ground us, among so many other things. Days punctuated with small, simple, and meaningful rituals help us to experience a greater presence of mind, body, and spirit, not to mention a sense of wholeness. You will be incorporating and integrating these rituals over time. When a ritual no longer serves, you will replace it with what *does* nourish your body and feed your soul at that present moment in time. Perhaps you will return to that ritual when it feels relevant again.

the rites of slow beauty: i am ready to receive

There is limitless energy within each of us, but it has been pummeled and buried by all of the distractions in our life, our inability to prioritize what is truly meaningful, and our blind spots when it comes to truly taking care of ourself in a sustainable way. At their core, rituals are a way of putting on our own oxygen mask before we attempt to take care of anyone else.

Here and now is where we put the Slow Beauty philosophy into practice.

In this chapter we will learn some strategies for slowing things down and returning to simplicity so that we can feel and express natural beauty in all of its facets: in our mind, in our body, and in our soul. Know that there isn't one specific route that will lead you to authentic beauty. The approach is a composite of mysticism, poetry, sensuality, meditation, nourishment, movement, conscious thinking, being present, being creative, emotional state, and even the language that we use. We each create our own composite and connect to it through the rituals we select to define our Slow Beauty practice. We are grounded in this internal place that expresses Slow Beauty through these rituals, which are intended to slow things down; calm the nervous system; promote intimacy and connectedness with ourself, others, and life itself; foster deeper sleep; provide greater strength; and allow us to both feel and look more energized and beautiful. Slow Beauty lends itself to such rituals because it is a graceful and calm beauty that represents the values of integrity, kindness, and trust—all of those values that have been undermined in our capitalistic society.

According to a study by World Value Survey conducted by Esteban Ortiz-Ospina and Max Roser, in the United States, interpersonal trust attitudes have decreased and people seem to trust one another less today than they did forty years ago. This is a meaningful—and sad—shift because, also according to the study, "Trust is a key contributor to sustainable well-being outcomes." Of course, this is true not only on national levels, but also in our own life. A Slow Beauty practice grounded in rituals will help us develop a deep and lasting sense of trust in both ourself and in the world we create.

Of course, the idea of beauty rituals is not new. But please understand that there is a big difference between beauty rituals and the beauty *regimes* that have been marketed to us. Slow Beauty is not a combination of natural products dressed in the same sexist, misogynistic imagery that pushes rigid beauty standards upon us. Any

movement—no matter how natural and holistic—that establishes standards is still showing us what beauty should be and how it should be attained. Slow Beauty is *your* unique perspective, *your* point of view about what it means to feel and look beautiful; not a photographer, designer, or editor's vision about what beautiful looks like. Each of us independently determines what beauty looks like—which means that beauty is inherently diverse, inclusive, expansive, creative, and ever-evolving. Always define your own fluid standard of beauty and ground yourself in it!

There is something peaceful about this Slow Beauty journey. It's bold kindness, rather than packing a shock value. It is quiet, unwavering strength that persists both in the calm and in the storm. When you develop that real intimacy and deep trust with yourself, your well-being is vastly enhanced. It will sometimes feel energetic, uplifting, and even ecstatic. This is because the rituals that you incorporate into your life are designed to remove any clots that have compromised the flow of your natural energy. They dissolve emotional and spiritual residue and that mental and physical plaque that keeps you in a state of status quo. The rituals keep our energy fluid and thus unstick those places where we are stuck. It's a beautiful thing, but also know that delving into these rituals involves a sort of self-initiation. Because of this, you may at times feel a bit lonely or it might be difficult to face aspects of yourself that are no longer serving you, to be able to bid them a final farewell as you become more invigorated and energized. This isn't always easy—but it *is* always worth it.

With these rituals comes the idea of energy. Everything around us is energy. Our goal is to tap into our natural rhythm, our own cadence, so as to align ourself with our personal wellspring of energy. When we don't have access to that energy, we feel weighed down because we are out of synch with our natural rhythm. For some of us, this might mean that we're spending too much time in our head and not enough time in our body or vice versa. For others it could mean that we're completely disconnected from our spirit or, conversely, so looped in to the spiritual realm that we're not grounded enough in our body. Or maybe your experience is entirely different. But the point here is to neutralize any combination that results in bringing us out of synch and cutting us off from our *prana*, our life force, our energetic flow.

The rituals create space for us to tap into the infinite, intuitive knowledge of our life force. When this energy is flowing naturally and without inhibition, miracles are possible. This free-flowing energy creates a fertile, fecund soil for the miracles to seed and come to life in all of their abundance, beauty, joy, love, strength, and wholeness. When we are closed, stagnant, judgmental, rigid, fixed, depressed, and exclusive, the soil is like a complete wasteland. Nothing can grow and develop and prosper—instead, there is death, disease, and fragmentation.

It is only when we are courageous enough to slow down—and, *yes*, this is an act of courage, particularly in today's society—that we will be able to move to our *own* rhythm rather than a rhythm or pace that is imposed upon us by someone else. Each one of us has our own unique rhythm and cadence. We should not judge whether we deem someone else's rhythm to be too fast or too slow but, rather, be open and accepting of everyone's rhythm. Maybe you don't even know what your own natural rhythm is. It is through the incorporation of these rituals that you will find out.

With some trial and error and a bit of experimentation, you will find which of the rituals in this section allow you to connect with your own life force and rhythm. Go into this process with the understanding that not all of these rituals will resonate with you. Experiment with them, build on them, evolve them, or simply walk away from any that you find don't correspond with your unique Slow Beauty practice. Remember as you try them on that you are looking for rituals—or for ways of performing and incorporating the rituals—that ground you in your inner pace, that bring you back to that pace when you are tempted to go off course, or that stave off any agenda that may be distracting you from your own personal map.

These rituals are also a form of self-empowerment. They are what empower you to reach beyond your current self and to achieve your better self. They will transport you to see and experience yourself and your life more expansively and with more vibrant energy. The rituals will help you identify and become the infinite, eternal self that you already are on the inside as opposed to identifying with the finite, external self that is compartmentalized by the expectations of others who tell you what you should and should not be doing.

You will find that incorporating these rituals into your life will shock your stagnated senses, overwhelming them with positivity and goodness. The space you've created will fill up with infor- mation and knowledge from your inner self. My best advice? Receive that information, whatever it looks like. And not only that, but receive it with *gratitude*. This information is nothing less than a gift for you to unwrap, experience, and enjoy.

Keep these words in mind as you embark on the journey of incorporating these rituals into your life: *I am honorable, I am holy, I am sacred. I am ready to receive.* You must learn how to receive well before you are able to give well. Get ready to receive lots of new, exciting information that will serve your mind, body, and soul as you begin to integrate these rituals into your own life!

know thyself

The rituals you'll find in the following pages are a collection of more than eighteen years of research and experimentation of various practices, pro- cesses, and ways of thinking as applied to mind, body, and soul. They've shaped my journey, and they have shaped me. More accurately, they *continue* to shape me as I revisit them over and over again. Each time we engage with a ritual we are in a unique place, in that moment, at that time. And thus we are able to revisit rituals over and over again, and always glean something new. That is the nature of rituals—they never get old. Rituals serve as touch points and doorways into the initiation of the mysteries of the self. They remove us from the din of the world and guide us into our personal sanctuary, a place of genuine and deep renewal. The rituals help us to better see and understand ourself, our relationships, and the world around us. In short, they help us to *know thyself.*

Rituals allow us to shed that which needs shedding, and to hunker down into that which requires grounding. They help us to share ourself when it's time to give, and to retreat when it's time for healing. The rituals give shape to the eternal natural cycles of birth and death, cycles that occur within and that we must connect with so as to live fluidly and with self-understanding. Much as a tree cannot resist the life cycles of the seasons, so too we must not resist the changing seasons within. In the winter we are bare, bearing witness—no matter how harsh the climate, we must see it with our own eye. In the spring we flower, in the summer we are full, and in fall we are changing and letting go. This is being in process—in *our* process of always becoming.

Many of these recommended rituals are just plain common sense—or, at least, they used to be. They used to be activities we seamlessly experienced in our life. Since the advent of technology and our subsequent reliance and addiction to it, we are moving further away from these once automatic health and wellness imperatives. Now we are required to make them intentional. Otherwise, we will lose the benefits they have to offer us. In a way, Slow Beauty is a plea to not allow these experiences to be pulled into the black hole of history and the long halls of our memory.

the real deal: seeing authentic beauty

Her name was Diotima, and she was a prophetess from ancient Greece who revealed the mysteries of love to Plato. In true Socratic style, they had intercourse (of the mind) wherein Diotima revealed the mysteries of love to Plato, and Plato, in turn, shared the insights he gleaned from Diotima in his famous text *Symposium*, the most renowned philosophical dialogue on the attributes of love ever created. Diotima's vision of love is that the pursuit of true love is really the pursuit of loving beauty;

it is the *form* of beauty. To help Plato understand her teachings on love, Diotima frames love as an ascent up a ladder. At the base of the ladder, she explains, exists the lustful loving of one body. Ascending up the ladder, the next rung is the understanding that all bodies are pretty much the same; with that comes the loving of all bodies (as in, "Love your neighbor as yourself"). From there, we ascend the ladder further to love the beauty of the soul. So, this ascension is an ascension from

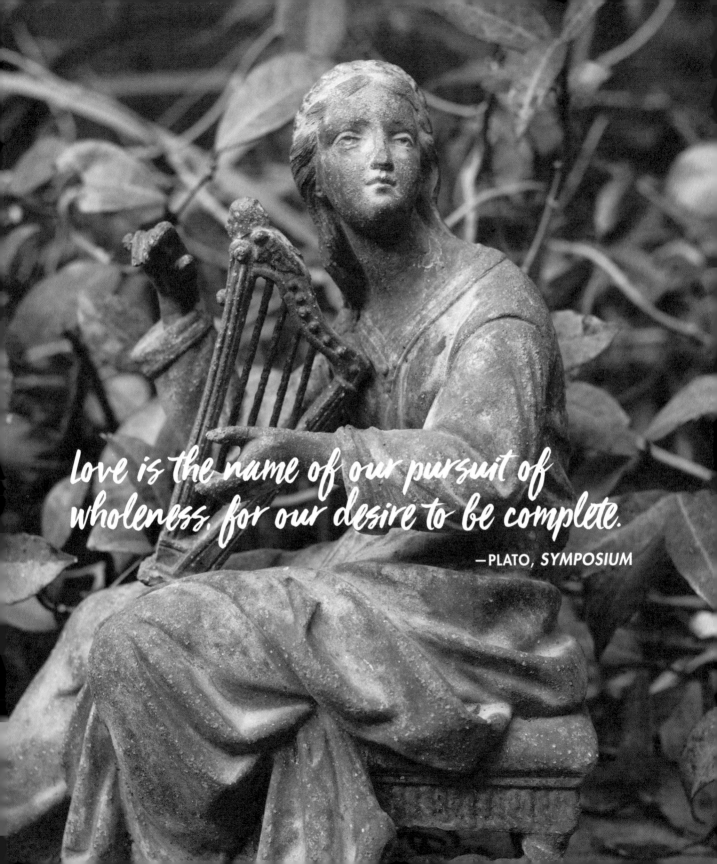

love is the name of our pursuit of wholeness, for our desire to be complete.

—PLATO, *SYMPOSIUM*

loving one particular body to "facing the vast sea of beauty" to loving beauty itself. That is, the type of beauty that only the soul can have.

In *Symposium,* Diotima describes beauty as "an everlasting loveliness, which neither comes nor goes, which neither flowers nor fades." It is the very essence of beauty, "subsisting of itself and by itself in an eternal oneness." She adds, "Those who are obsessed with images of beauty can only produce images of virtue, but those who can see Beauty itself can produce virtue itself, making themselves immortal and loved by the gods."

as above, so below: the spiritualization of beauty

Beauty is inherently spiritual, although that certainly isn't what is being reflected in the imagery of beauty being sold to us. The beauty we see in our culture today exists on the lowest rung of Diotima's ladder and has undertones (not to mention overtones) of pornography, violence, sexism, and misogyny. People have been railing against how women are being portrayed in the media and in advertising for years—yet, still, nothing has changed. In fact, according to Jean Kilbourne, gender expert for women's rights who has been at the forefront of this dialogue for forty years, nothing has changed. In fact, she has said that it has actually gotten worse.

We've all heard the maxim "As above, so below," but what does it really mean? I believe that when we boil it down, it means this: There is the entire universe outside of us and there is an entire universe within us. Today, we are hyperfocused on the external universe—we explore it, study it, categorize it, dissect it, analyze it, innovate it, design it, interrelate in it, theorize about it, contemplate it, love it, disrespect it, are in awe of it, and so on and so on, ad infinitum. But what about the inner universe? This is the new frontier. The fact that yoga and meditation have infiltrated the Western mind is a happy sign that we are ready to explore this new frontier.

Our recent discoveries about the plasticity and neurodiversity of the brain, the explosion of interest in neuroscience, and our increased comfort level with exploring virtual worlds through our smartphones and tablets (metaphorically "leaving" one reality to explore another) are all telltale signs that we are poised and ready to take this deep dive into the vast universe of the self. We're ready to focus on designing our interior life just as we design our exterior life.

If we pay closer attention to the design of our inner life—to our thoughts and emotions, to feeding our soul, and taking care of our body so that it can operate optimally—then we may be able to align our internal and external realities to be matched, complete, and whole. Our mind, body, and soul do not operate separately; they operate as a whole. What affects one part has an effect on the other parts, for better or for worse. How we orient ourself internally is what will be reflected back to us externally. The world is like a mirror reflecting what is going on internally. If you are seeing things in that mirror that do not feel right, that means there is work to be done by *you*.

We will use these rituals to help us to get the work done. When we are busy and distracted all of the time, it's because we don't want to do the work, because we are avoiding the real work. This is where we come back to that idea of having the courage to slow down so that we are able to create a true reflection of beauty. I'm not telling you anything you don't already know—all of this knowledge is within you. You have just been buried in biases and distractions and procrastinations and a lack of self-trust. This busyness is a compulsion; it is a fear of facing the unknown authentic self because the home has been neglected for so long that there is an emptiness, a *horror vacui* that is difficult to wrestle with and to come to terms with. There really is no other way but to face that emptiness and wrestle with it.

Rituals help us wake up and breathe life into the dusty, forgotten, overlooked, neglected areas of our internal self. They shed light through our dusty windows, and bring warmth to the interior rooms. They help us to remember our knowledge, our wisdom, our beauty. Rituals are remembering in motion. The only catch? Remembering isn't always easy. As you wake up, you will come to understand the abuses, the compromises, and the passive-aggressive relationship you have been having with yourself. It will hurt you, and as your old self dies, you will experience grief. Let it come, don't fight it. Use the rituals to help you through it. The rituals are designed to help you become radically compassionate with yourself so you will become radically compassionate with others. Once you make this renewed commitment to truly love and respect yourself, there is no turning back.

what's my story?

Each of us has a running narrative about who we are and where we've been. It's usually connected to our upbringing, the roles we play, and the masks we wear. Sometimes we share that narrative with others. Often, we don't even realize we are locked into a particular narrative.

Let's take a while here to become aware of our internal narrative and to make sure it is working for us—that it is supportive, nourishing, and expansive. If we find there are aspects that are not serving us, then we need to rework these parts and do some editing.

Before I was asked this question myself, I had never really thought about my story. It wasn't until I began the long process of thinking my narrative through and identifying the gaps, heartaches, and blessings that I started to weave together a more cohesive story. In the ensuing years, I've found this ritual is particularly helpful for those who have suffered from trauma.

RITUAL:
REWRITE YOUR STORY

Imagine how freeing changing up your story can be. You've been carrying this narrative around with you from the very beginning of your life. It's a story you have told yourself over and over again, as if it were a broken record. A story so ingrained in your essence, so known, so comfortable, so much like a second skin that you are the living, breathing expression of that story. You enact and reenact this story every single day of your life, in all of your interactions, relationships, body movements, facial expressions, speech patterns, postures, styles, and food choices.

If you are perfectly content with all of the aspects of your storyline, then you can stop reading now. If you're not, then keep on going. We're about to refine those aspects of your storyline that are not supporting you, sustaining you, making you feel beautiful, or that are keeping you from growing young. Wherever you are right now in your heroine journey, you have the opportunity to acknowledge the path you are on and to either choose to continue on that same path, or to make a new, different choice. Or, even better yet, you can create a narrative that serves as a map. It is by creating this map that you will obtain the biggest picture and the best perspective. This is what I mean by always *becoming*.

Oftentimes, it takes some kind of large event to cast us out to a new adventure, away from the known, comfortable, status quo roles we have taken on. It is when the routine of our life gets challenged and from those things that may feel stressful, confusing, or challenging that we find those life-affirming silver linings that provide us with an opportunity for growth. These are the paradoxes life hides and holds for us. The gifts are wrapped inside of the paradoxes. Within those very life experiences that appear senseless and meaningless is often buried an inner truth ripe with meaning and offering depth and growth potential. It is in that liminal state between the old way of knowing and the potential of the new way that the truth is often revealed. This requires patience and the ability to have the courage to slow down, to live with ambiguity for a while, to make time for that reflection so that we can uncover the truth and integrate it into our process of self-actualization. Major life events often offer us this opportunity through the form of unexpected wakeup calls.

But, outside of these turning-point moments and experiences that we can't conjure up, there is a way to slow down and experience self-reflective moments each and every day. You guessed it: rituals. Rituals arrest that status quo state of mind and help us gain a new perspective that allows us to see ourself in a new, refreshing light.

This is a time to discard any notions you might have that new perspectives, stories, and views of the self are only for the young. We are always evolving, always growing, and, in particular, always growing younger. No matter what chapter of life you're in right now, you always get to write the next one. Our stories are not confined by any sort of boundaries, including age limits.

So, with this ritual, your exercise is to share your story with someone. It might be a trusted friend, your partner, or even a stranger. Share your story with them, paying equal attention to what you share and what you omit. Note how they respond. Note the feelings and thoughts that come up, both as you are sharing the story and after. And then think about your edit. If you have been telling yourself a story that is resulting in harsh, negative thoughts about yourself, then this is a way to get to the roots of the issue, and to pull those roots out! This is an opportunity to tell your story in a more life-affirming manner, with a refreshing, loving perspective. You may even want to consider recording yourself as you tell this story so that you can come back to it later and see how your story has evolved over time.

finding sanctuary and designing your inner life

For thousands of years, man has been building sacred structures around the world for people to enter and experience an awe intended to humble. We call these structures sanctuaries. They come in the form of our great pyramids, grand churches, and impressive temples. Every culture expresses itself through its unique architecture. Inside of the thick walls of these inviting sanctuaries, worshipers and seekers are enraptured by a special variety of quietness. They are, quite literally, a sanctuary from the chaos and distractions of the outside world. Whatever takes place outside is held at bay to provide the opportunity to slowly experience something more profound, more poetic, deeper, and more sacred. Inside of these sanctuaries, time stands still as we experience beauty—slow beauty. When we stand inside of these places, we are really a sanctuary standing within a sanctuary, because we are also our very own sanctuaries. We are the embodiment of the sanctuary. It's just that outside, amid all of the chaos and distraction, this can be more difficult to see.

When we enter the structures, we do so with respect. Since we, too, are sanctuaries, this is also how we should be within ourself. We wake up full of life every day and, really, what is more sacred than this?

Rituals can help us show our inner sanctuary the same respect we show these brick and mortar sanctuaries. We demonstrate this respect for our own sanctuaries in the form of thinking good thoughts, surrounding ourself with loving people, offering ourself the right food, pleasure, good conversation, movement, and creative expression. Just as temples and churches have been designed as a safe space to express our deepest desires and needs, so too must our inner life be designed. We, too, contain what is holy. With this, we must also think about who we allow to access our personal sanctuary. Who would you like to be a member of your temple? We do not grow by isolating ourself from others, but our growth can also be slowed down or halted altogether if we spend time with people who are not aligned with our values and our needs. So, be discerning. This is, after all, our temple—and we are completely in charge of how we would like to design it.

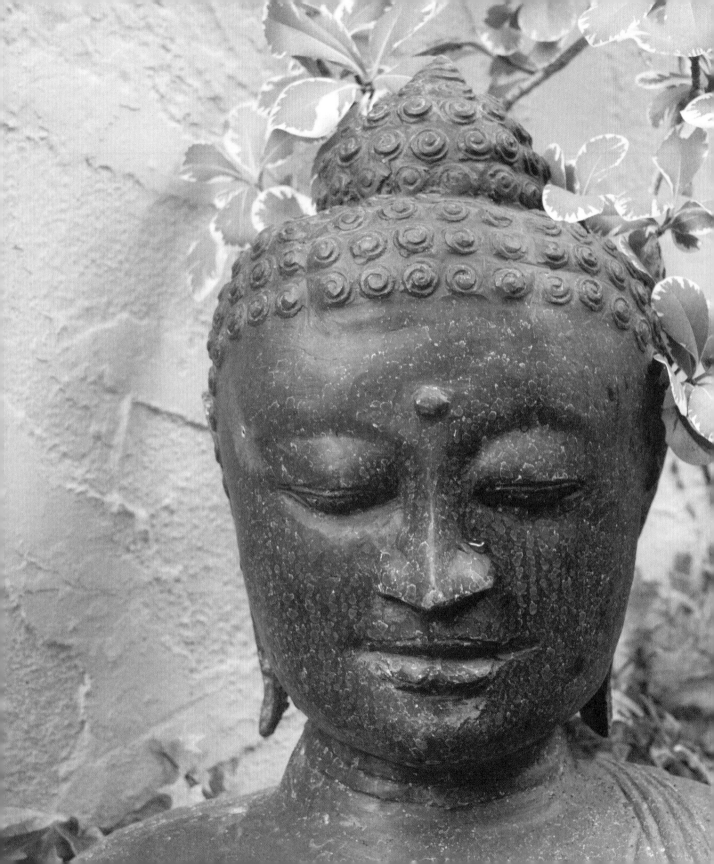

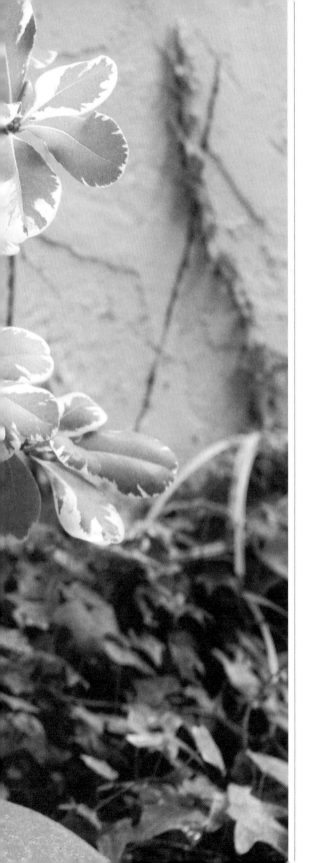

RITUAL:
YOUR INNER TEMPLE

Through this interactive experiential visualization, we will make space for ourself by designing our very own temple. With this, we want to think about the lighting, the music, the scent, the décor, the layout, the materials, the height of the ceiling, the language used inside the temple, the sound, the feelings, the tastes—all of those things that come to mind when you think about a sacred space. We are going analog. This is a "slower times" type of exercise. Take out your markers, magazines, scissors, tape, glue, and whatever else you need to create your vision of your very own inner sanctuary. Create it right here in this book, on these pages. There are blank pages at the end. If you need more space, then let it spill over into other areas of the book. You can even cover up words if need be. Most important, free yourself to create—no judgment, no perfection, just get your vision onto the page. It can and should be both aspects of what works for you and what is aspirational. You can work in drafts, feeling free to revisit, edit, and build upon your temple.

Once you have created a vision of your inner temple, you'll find that you carry it with you everywhere. Perhaps you will want to share what you've created with others and maybe not. When I received my own personal meditation mantra from my teacher many years ago, I was advised not share it with others, to keep it sacred, so that it became wholly my own. You might want to apply this same philosophy to the visual of your inner temple. After all, it *is* sacred.

What you're creating here is a visual version of your inner temple. Your very own special place, to be visited over and over again. A place where your innermost self resides. Entertain the thought that, over time, you will grow to need a new temple. When you feel that need arising, honor it and then take the steps to remodel and rebuild. Move the furniture around, break down the walls, bust through the ceilings, expand, invite new people in, change the programming. Evolve. Always be evolving.

NOTE TO SELF

It is especially difficult to find the right words to describe something as subtle and nuanced as the inner life. Throughout this book, I mention a union *with* the self and *of* the self many times over. The idea of self and the inner life is so abstract that it can be tempting to give up on this quest, to live in clichés, or to remain unsure if all of this work of becoming we are doing is actually paying off.

When we think of that ultimate inner connection, that coming home to self, and renewing of the self, it's worth noting how the Buddha referenced "self" as "no-self." It's a paradox, a riddle, a treasure hunt. With this in mind, it's actually the disappearance of the "self" that we seek, and it arrives in glimpses, in breezes. It is like a presence of the absence of the self. This type of presence has been described as feelings of bliss, oneness, or enlightenment. I describe it as a kind of softening, or a more organic shape of feelings and thoughts. When they're too rigid, feelings and thoughts have the ability to paralyze our growth. They inhibit and stifle our need to be spontaneous, open-minded, flexible, and creative. We get stuck in a concrete storyline instead of one that is fluid, infinite, and eternal. On the other hand, we touch eternity when the presence of the absence of the self is present.

In Kabbalah this idea of "no-self" is known as *tzimtzum*, and is told in the context of the creation myth. It is described as a withdrawal: God created the world and then withdrew, thus allowing the world to create itself out of the elements that God had introduced—light, water, plants, grass, seeds, sun, moon, stars, fish, birds, humans, and a day of rest.

In this line of thinking, withdrawal occurs to provide an opportunity for independence to develop. And so it is with self and the inner life. We need to provide opportunities of withdrawal from the stressful life we live so as to allow space for our inner life to develop, grow, and prosper. We need independence and these moments of separation from our self (from our roles, our responsibilities, and our masks) to create a stronger sense of self. In the largest sense, Slow Beauty is showing you ways to stand not apart from, but *alongside* yourself and to bear witness to life's miraculous unfolding.

the big share:
we're stronger together

Speaking of sacred spaces that call to mind various religions, it seems like a good time to bring up this point: While Slow Beauty does not promote any sort of specific religious dogma, I do believe that, when blended together, ancient practices and techniques will give us the strongest, most expansive experience. Maybe we were culturally fractioned for a reason, and now is the time to come together as one big community—one *human* community of sharing, caring, trusting, loving, learning, thriving, and kindness. That's the world I want to live in. I'm going to believe in and work toward that until the day I die. I'm committed to this belief. Are you?

So, yes, we are a broken world. We are fragmented, both personally and universally. Perhaps this social fragmentation is a critical part of our evolutionary process. I know it's kind of a sci-fi musing, but it's an amusing thought, if nothing else. Now is the time for us to pick up our various pieces and meld them back together. We don't discard, we carefully, mindfully, and compassionately put it all back together again—and we do this *together*. It's a paradox, the perfection of imperfection. Think back to that Japanese concept of kintsigu, the art of repairing objects that break rather than discarding them. I would argue that this concept is very much needed in this age of cheap, disposable, easily discarded objects. Kintsigu treats the breakage and repair of an object as a part of the history of that object, something to be highlighted and illuminated, rather than disguised.

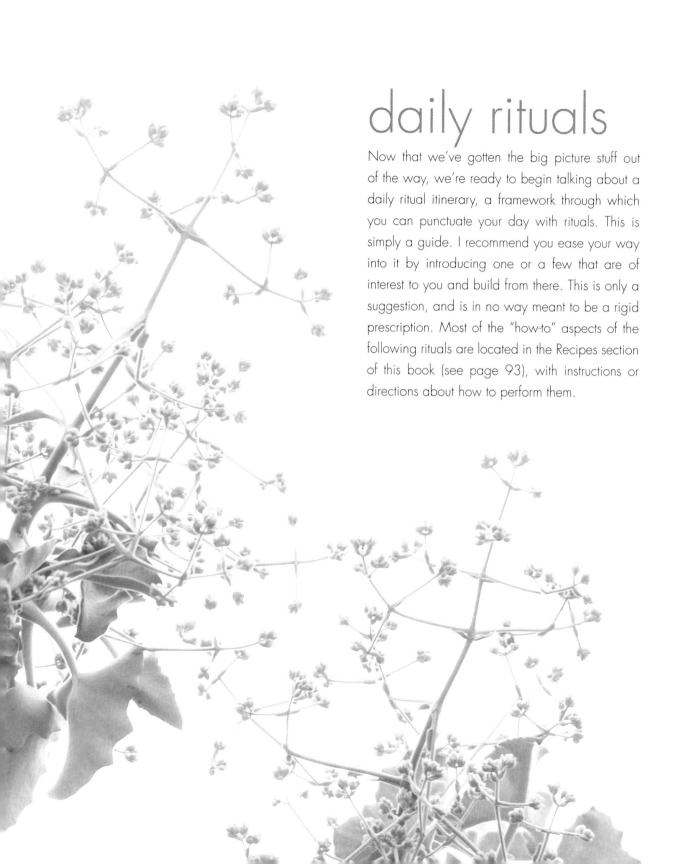

daily rituals

Now that we've gotten the big picture stuff out of the way, we're ready to begin talking about a daily ritual itinerary, a framework through which you can punctuate your day with rituals. This is simply a guide. I recommend you ease your way into it by introducing one or a few that are of interest to you and build from there. This is only a suggestion, and is in no way meant to be a rigid prescription. Most of the "how-to" aspects of the following rituals are located in the Recipes section of this book (see page 93), with instructions or directions about how to perform them.

first light

The goal here is to bring our circadian rhythm back in line with nature by triggering melatonin. This simple act both energizes us and regularizes our sleep patterns, which is nothing short of critical to beauty and good health.

First Light is something I look forward to each morning when I wake up. In fact, it's the very first thing I do every morning. It's as simple as this: I get out of bed, go downstairs, open the door, and step outside to feel the natural light. Of course, this is easier to do in the spring and summer months when the temperature is warmer and the sunlight is available earlier. If you wake up early in the fall and winter months, chances are it is still dark outside. In this case, I still walk outside for the fresh air, but I do so when the light becomes available.

WHY IT WORKS

Each of us has an internal master clock called a circadian clock. This clock works in twenty-four-hour cycles, and it regulates the physiological processes in the body as well as signaling us when it's time to sleep. This body clock responds to environmental cues, such as light, darkness, and temperature. Located in the hypothalamus, it is made up of two clusters of thousands of nerve cells. Exposure to natural light first thing in the morning helps reset our body clock, which assists the processes of our natural internal rhythm in working optimally.

WHY DO IT?

Light in the morning helps us wake up. It energizes us and helps jump-start the production of melatonin to promote a good night's sleep when the time comes. It may sound counterintuitive to start producing the hormone that makes us sleepy as we wake up, but we need to build up enough melatonin throughout the course of the day to ensure a good night's sleep. Adequate amounts of light affect our sleeping patterns, productivity, alertness, and mood. It also improves our metabolic function. So, let the light in. Let the light shine on you.

HOW TO DO IT

Go outside first thing in the morning and look at the natural light. Also note that Third Light is important for all of the same reasons, but in reverse. Dim your interior lights at least one hour before bedtime. This signals you that it's time to go to sleep and have a good night's rest.

Ideally, we want to spend a combined amount of at least one hour outdoors per day.

morning meditation

A morning meditation is a great ritual for starting off the day with an intentional connection with yourself. Checking in with ourself prior to beginning a hectic day full of unknown surprises grounds us in calmness and aids us in dealing with the ebbs and flows of the day ahead. Meditation is not meant for us to try to control our thoughts; rather, it is a tool to help us understand that thoughts come and go. (For more on meditation, see page 166.)

morning movement

By the time we start our day, our body has been at rest in a prone state for many hours. Often we don't have time to make it to a morning exercise or yoga class. Morning Movement is a ritual to get the blood flowing and remind us that we have a body that needs our attention. It is an opportunity to rejoice in and be grateful for the body in which we reside. Toning, opening, stretching, strengthening, and releasing are some of the benefits of Morning Movement. (See page 173 for seasonally appropriate body movements.)

morning exfoliation

Exfoliation is a deep cleanse for the skin. In-shower skin exfoliation stimulates the lymph nodes, removes dead skin cells, tones the skin, and awakens the senses. It eliminates toxins and clears the mind; it breaks down fatty tissues, and helps reduce the appearance of age spots on the skin. It helps prevent ingrown hairs, reduces stress, and because it increases blood circulation, it also creates glowing, healthy skin.

HOW TO DO IT

Work morning exfoliation into your regular shower routine two or three times per week. In the shower, wet your entire body and then place an ample amount of sugar scrub in your hand. Beginning at the bottom of your feet and working your way up, massage a seasonal scrub (see page 149) all over your body, using a circular motion with gentle, even pressure on all areas except for the rougher areas (such as the knees and elbows), which require a firmer pressure. Exfoliate from left to right over your belly so that you are in sync with the natural flow of your digestion. Once you reach the midsection of your body around your heart, continue upward around your chest, paying special attention to your thorax with a bit of extra pressure and then move on to your neck, still using that circular motion. (Please note these instructions are for wet sugar-scrubbing. There are recipes for two dry sugar scrubs and the instructions are in the Recipes section, on page 150.)

Once you've opened your pores with exfoliation, massage oil (see page 156) over your body to nourish the skin. Remember to drink extra amounts of water on the days you exfoliate because you are encouraging new skin cells and you want them to be nourished from the inside out.

morning self-massage

The skin is the largest organ of the body and it needs to be touched. Touch triggers the feel-good hormone oxytocin, decreases anxiety, and lowers blood pressure, among so many other benefits. *

Because our skin is porous, it absorbs many of the ingredients we put on it, so it is important that we use products that contain natural and organic ingredients whenever possible. Self-massage is excellent for overall health and well-being, reduces anxiety, calms the nerves, lubricates the joints, tones skin and makes it soft and smooth, improves and deepens sleep, increases circulation, improves mental alertness, nourishes the skin and tissues, and allows toxins to be released from the body.

*"5 Reasons to Make Time for Cuddling" by Ysolt Usigan, *Shape*, http://www.shape.com/lifestyle/sex-and-love/5-health-reasons-make-time-cuddling.

HOW TO DO IT

For the morning self-massage, I've included a variation on the traditional Ayurvedic self-massage known as *ahbyanga*. This variation should be practiced postshower daily, using a light amount of oil, which will remain on the skin after you've massaged.

If you'd like to try a more extended version of this massage in the evening, you can also include your scalp, keeping the oil in your hair overnight, and apply a heavier amount of oil on your skin. The evening version of this massage is recommended a few times per week in the cooler seasons and one time per week in warmer seasons. Most important, this massage should be done intentionally. As you perform the massage, massage not only the oil blends into your skin but also think loving, supportive, and nourishing thoughts. This massage is a wonderful opportunity to become more accepting of your body. Use one of your DIY mantras (see page 167) during this time.

(1) Warm the oil, either by running hot water over the bottle or in your hands. Use about 1 tablespoon of oil, or just enough that it will seep into your skin. This is intended to be a light oil massage so you can put on your clothes after without staining the clothing.

(2) Gently massage your face and ears, paying special attention to your temples and behind and under your ears. Use the tip of your finger to apply a couple of drops of oil to the opening of your ear canal.

(3) Massage the front and back of your neck, using an open palm to create friction.

(4) Massage your arms, using a circular motion at your shoulders and elbows, and back-and-forth motions on your upper arms and forearms.

(5) Massage your chest and stomach, using a straight up-and-down motion over your breastbone, and a gentle clockwise circular motion over your abdomen. Come back up to your thorax region (your heart and lungs) and apply an extra clockwise circular motion with a bit of extra pressure.

(6) Apply a bit of oil to both of your hands, then gently reach around to your back and spine, massaging up and down as well as you can without straining.

(7) Massage your legs vigorously, using circular motions at your ankles and knees, and back-and- forth motions on your shins, calves, hamstrings, and thighs.

(8) Spend extra time on your feet. Massage back-and-forth over the soles of your feet and toes, using the open part of your hand.

(9) Keep a thin film of oil on your body as it is beneficial for toning your skin and warming your muscles throughout the day.

* The steps above are guidelines on how to approach self-massage. As you become more proficient, listen to your body's needs, applying more pressure or paying more attention to parts of your body that require more love. This self-massage should gradually become a personalized, intuitive technique addressing your specific needs. When you slow down, you are better able to tune into what those needs are.

IN THE AFTERNOON ——————————————

solar light

Just like morning, solar noon is also an optimal time to get some light exposure. If you are at the office, step outside and let the light shine on you. If you are able, twenty minutes is ideal.

afternoon meditation

Several hours into your day is a good time to release some of the stress that has built up. Afternoon meditation provides an opportunity to keep the stress from building up too much, and gives you a time-out from whatever the day is demanding of you. This meditation might be in the form of a traditional meditation technique (see page 167), time spent in nature, a nap, or any other activity that you find calming. You may feel as if you are too busy for this time-out. Let me tell you this: Taking this time for yourself will actually help you be more productive for the rest of the day. *

afternoon movement

We spend so much of our daily life sitting down. This is such an extreme condition that you've probably heard "sitting is the new smoking." Afternoon Movement helps alleviate this by reminding you to get out of your seat, wherever you are, and to move around a bit. Starting on page 173, you'll find a variety of movements that are easily done anywhere, anytime, no special clothing required.

afternoon mist

A seasonal spritz of mist to the face is a great afternoon pick-me-up. The mist will rehydrate and refresh your skin. Not only that, but each seasonal mist (found starting on page 161) includes specific beneficial ingredients to uplift your mind, body, and spirit.

*David Levy, "The Effects of Mindfulness Meditation Training on Multitasking in a High-Stress Information Environment," University of Washington, 2012, http://faculty.washington.edu/wobbrock/pubs/gi-12.02.pdf.

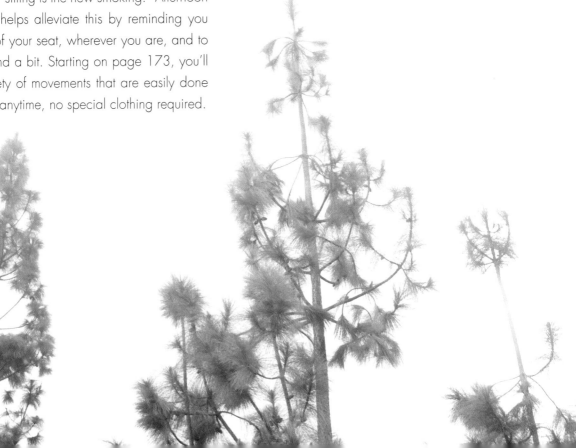

third light

About an hour before bedtime, begin to dim the lights in the house to encourage your body to prepare for sleep.

evening meditation

Right before bedtime is a good time to do a gratitude meditation. You can do this lying down, by simply thinking about everything you are grateful for from the day as you drift off to sleep. Or you can keep a daily gratitude journal and write down all the things you are grateful for.

I do the Heart Belly breathing meditation where I place one hand on my heart and one hand on my belly and I breath in and out through my nose until my thoughts slow down.

evening movement

Intentional movements prior to bed will help you release some of the toxins and stress you have collected from your day and help support a good night's rest. See page 173 for some specific suggestions.

evening self-massage

This self-massage is meant to apply a warm, thick layer of oil to your skin, almost like a blanket, to help calm anxiety and worry. Try it three times per week. Warm ½ cup of massage oil (see page 156). Spread the oil evenly over your body, waiting a few minutes before you start massaging it in, to allow the oil to be absorbed into your skin.

Massage your body from bottom to top, using the same technique used for Morning Self-Massage (page 63) and also allowing it to evolve into intuitive touch over time. Use a firm, even pressure over all areas of your body, except for sensitive spots, such as your heart and abdomen, where you will use a lighter pressure. For such areas as the soles of your feet, the palms of your hands, and the base of your fingernails (in other words, those areas where the nerve endings are more concentrated), use more oil and spend more time massaging. Leave the oil on overnight to allow it to deeply penetrate the skin and connective tissues. I recommend keeping a robe or an old pair of pajamas on hand specifically for this occasion because the oil may stain.

Finish by massaging your scalp. Begin with a dry, circular massage around your hairline. Then disperse a tablespoon of oil onto your scalp and hair. Beginning at the front of your hairline and working your way toward the back, use your fingertips to massage the oil into your entire scalp, using deep, slow movements. Repeat this sequence three to four times, then end with a hair tug. Wrap your head in a towel for ten minutes or leave it on overnight.

In the morning, rinse off the oil in the shower and shampoo it out of your hair.

evening foot wash and massage

When my grandmother came to visit me when I was a child, she would always soak and wash my feet in the bathroom sink, then massage them before I went to bed. An evening foot wash and massage is so soothing—especially if you spend a lot of time on your feet or wear high heels. My grandmother taught me this from a young age.

To begin, fill up your sink, bathtub, or a large bowl with warm water. Place 1 cup of magnesium salts into the water, plus 2 to 3 drops of your favorite essential oil. Mix until the salts dissolve. Sit back and relax as you soak your feet in the water for 10 to 15 minutes. Remove your feet from the water and towel them dry.

To massage, pour 1 teaspoon (per foot) of your seasonal oil (page 156) into your hands, then rub your hands together to warm the oil. Place each hand on either side of your foot and, beginning at the toes and moving toward the

heel, rub the oil into your foot, being sure to rub it in between your toes. Pay special attention to rough, dry areas, such as your heels. End by rubbing the oil into your ankle in a circular motion.

Place your foot on your opposite thigh to access the bottom of the foot. We're going to perform some reflexology, which is massaging pressure points to stimulate different areas of the central nervous system. All the toes are associated with the head and neck, so massaging this area is known to secrete melatonin, which aids in a better night's sleep and releases tension in the neck and shoulders.

Using your thumb, inch up each toe, making sure to massage the top of each toe as well as the sides. Once you've reached the top of your toes, work your way back down again. Next, use your thumb to massage up and down the inner side of your foot. This area is associated with the spine. Now move your thumb to press the ball of your foot, which is associated with the chest. This will help calm and deepen your breath. Massage under the ball of your foot to promote feelings of deep relaxation, and then move to your heel. Press softly here a few times to foster a restful sleep. The bottom of the heel is associated with the sciatica nerve, and there is an insomnia point just at the top, center point of the heel. To finish, moisturize your foot, and then run another layer of oil over the foot. Put on a sock to lock in the moisture. Repeat these steps on the opposite foot.

evening nail care

Healthy cuticles equal healthy nails. Do not cut your cuticles, but instead apply cuticle oil to your nails daily to prevent hangnails and keep your nails hydrated. Because we use our hands so much, our nails are prone to drying, splitting, and peeling. Much of this is also related to our diet, and, of course, a whole balanced diet is always recommended, but a good cuticle oil can also do wonders.

In the evening, use your seasonal oil (section found on page 156) to hydrate your nails. Place a drop on each nail of your hands and feet and massage the oil into your cuticle. Not only will this hydrate your nails, but they'll also look shiny and healthy. Healthy cuticles promote healthy nail growth.

Since each of the seasonal oils contains fragrant essential oils, I find it's nice to begin this ritual with a breathing exercise. Before your apply the oil to your cuticles, cup your hands over your nose and mouth and breathe in deeply through your nose to the count of six; exhale for six. Repeat three times and notice your body relaxing and letting go.

THROUGHOUT THE DAY
drink your water

Chances are, this isn't news to you, but it's important to hear and practice it: Drink plenty of water. We all know this, but too often we don't remember to actually do it. The general rule of thumb is that you want to drink eight 8-ounce glasses of water a day. You also need to take into account your sex, body weight, environment, how active you are, and your health. My recommendation? Talk with your doctor to get a personalized water prescription based on all of these factors.

In addition to drinking regular, still water, I like to infuse my waters with muddled ingredient blends that offer further nourishment. I choose blends seasonally so as to tap into the rich resources available to us in the rhythm and timing of when nature produces it. The selection of ingredients and preparation of these water-based elixirs produces a state of multisensory mindfulness—touching the ingredients, seeing their colors, and breathing in their scent as you muddle them elevates our state of mind. This is a subtle thing, to be sure, but it is these slow, subtle ritual infusions that assuage our mind, body, and soul. The distinct taste adds another potent value to it, as well as the benefits of each of the active ingredients you are ingesting. (See page 139 for a listing of suggested water infusions.)

WHY DO IT?

Water flushes the toxins out from our vital organs and it carries nutrients to our cells. It also provides a moist environment for the tissues of our ears, nose, and throat. Even a low level of dehydration can reduce energy levels, which makes us feel tired. We lose fluids in a variety of ways, so it's important to remember to replenish our water supply by drinking water and/or eating foods that contain it, such as watermelon, strawberries, cantaloupe, grapefruit, cucumber, lettuce, radishes, and celery.

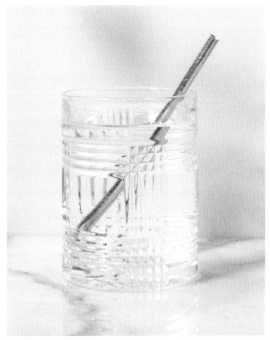

take some tea time

Japanese tea ceremonies involve four key principles known as "the way of tea": harmony, respect, purity, and tranquility. Japanese tea ceremonies consist of intentional steps and procedures to help guests slow down and experience tea as a multisensory meditative experience. The processes and procedures are detailed, intentional, and impart a sense of calm.

I recommend enjoying the appropriate seasonal tea (page 106) as you incorporate tea into your day. Creating a tea ritual for yourself is a way to be present, calm the central nervous system, and experience a sense of well-being and renewal. Make the tea ceremony a practice in being present by boiling your tea in an electric or old-fashioned teakettle and selecting a special teacup that is aesthetically pleasing to you. Be intentional about selecting a shape, color, and size that you love.

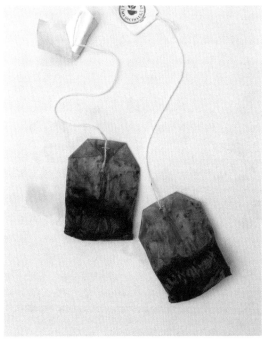

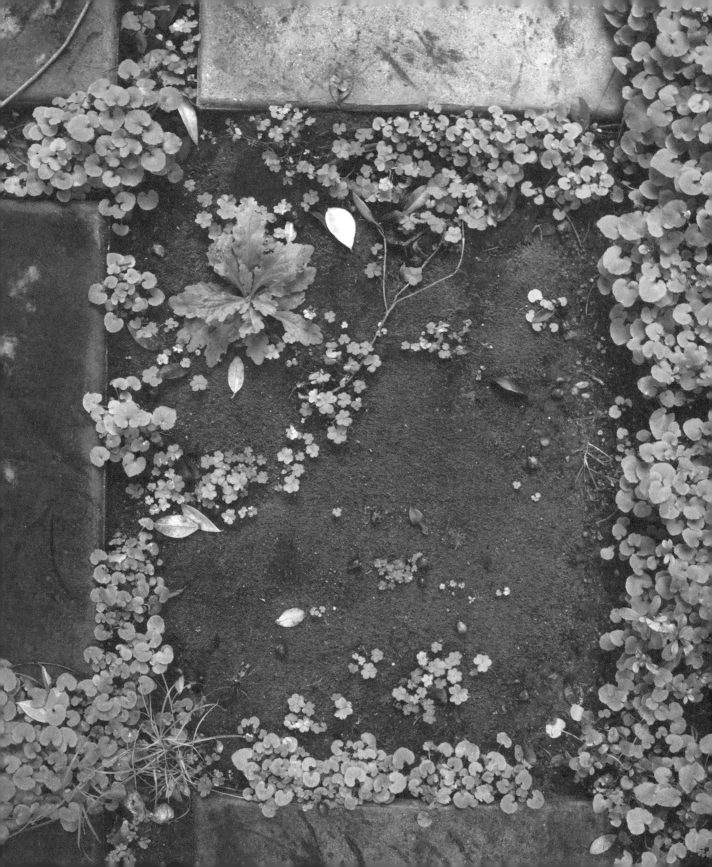

weekly, monthly, or yearly rituals

These rituals may be incorporated into your Slow Beauty practice on a daily, weekly, monthly, or yearly basis. Select from the following list and work them into your Mapping (see page 187) as it feels natural.

nature bathing

In his book *Earthing* (2010), Clinton Ober highlights all the benefits of immersing ourself in nature, such as reducing the stress-producing hormone cortisol, inflammation, and muscle tension; improving sleep; and increasing energy. I know that when I spend time soaking in nature, my entire mood lifts. This is not necessarily a momentary benefit, either. Depending on the amount of time I spend communing with the great outdoors, I may feel that lift reverberating throughout my life for days to come.

A recent Nielsen audience report revealed that adults spend over ten hours per day in front of a screen—and that number is growing. This accounts for nearly half of our day. If we spend eight hours sleeping, that leaves us with only six hours of nonscreen time each day. This is alarming, and it's important that we remember it hasn't always been this way. As a child of the '80s, I would often walk home from school, then while away the hours before dinner climbing trees, running, or biking around the neighborhood. Even in the midst of frigid Michigan winters, I would bundle up in a snowsuit and spend hours outside breaking icicles off of the side of my house to use for the snow forts I built.

Experiences like mine are quickly becoming a thing of the past as the world changes rapidly. There is now even a condition called nature-deficit disorder, a term coined by Richard Louv in his book *Last Child in the Woods*. He cites the "lure of the screen" as one of the main culprits in bringing about this disorder. Less exposure to nature is linked to depression, anxiety, and challenges handling stress.

Nature bathing provides us with a way to immerse ourself in nature. The idea here is to spend at least thirty minutes per day outside, with your bare feet on the ground, reconnecting to earth. Too often today, we treat nature as if it is a stranger—we fear it, label it, and avoid it. The truth is, we are only robbing ourself. Being in nature is so healing for the mind, body, and soul.

Look deep into nature and then you will understand everything better.

—ALBERT EINSTEIN

Seek out daily opportunities to connect with nature. The first and second light sequence is one way to make that connection because it gets you outdoors immediately upon waking, and away from your desk again at midday. More important, carve out time to really immerse yourself in nature for extended periods of time. Ideally, this time will also be disconnected time—allow yourself the freedom of unplugging.

In addition to walking outside, find time for such activities as hiking, camping, and biking. Your outdoor adventure can be either challenging or meandering, depending upon what you need that particular day. One of my favorite days in recent memory was spent on a ropes course with my kids. The course was in the middle of a forest, so we were exposed to the trees, fresh air, and three-dimensionality of the woods, as we used our body to traverse the courses. Being high up in the trees, focusing on my next balanced step, served as a form of deep meditation. I was breathing deeply, and fully present in the now. I felt the ben-

efits for days afterward! It elevated my mood and cleared my mind of racing thoughts.

The amount of time we spend away from nature, whether it be in our house, office, or car, is an act of self-imposed cruelness. We were not designed to sit in cubicles like barn animals (barn animals are not meant to be there, either). The entire office environment needs to be rethought and nature brought into the design. The same can be said about our learning institutions. Children spend way too much time stuck behind closed doors in classrooms, cut off from the environment they are meant to explore and be curious and open-minded about. We need to find more ways to bring nature closer to us so we are not estranged from (and even worse, fear) the beauty and benefits of nature where we can savor silence, reconnect with our authentic self, and benefit from the healing medicine of being immersed in nature.

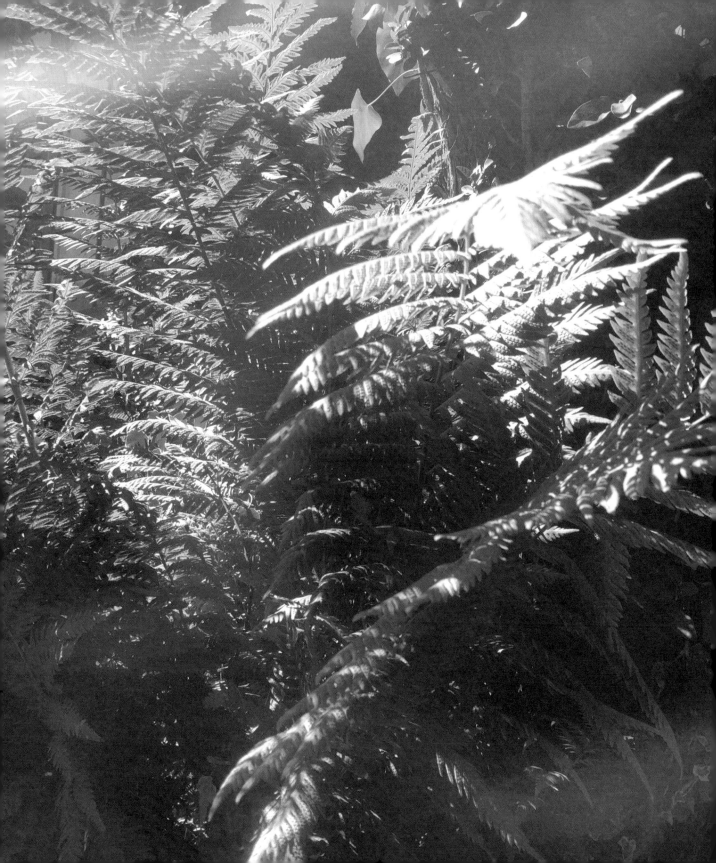

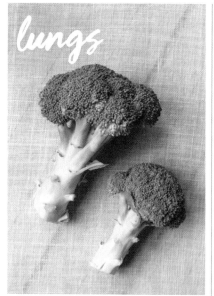

lungs

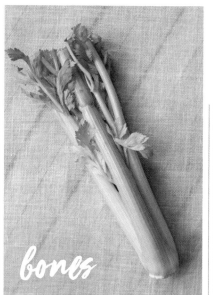

bones

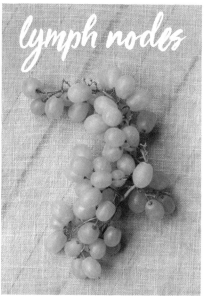

lymph nodes

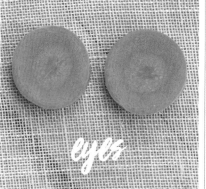

eyes

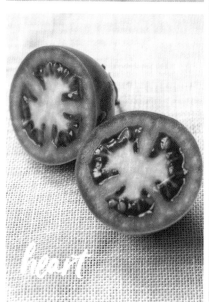

heart

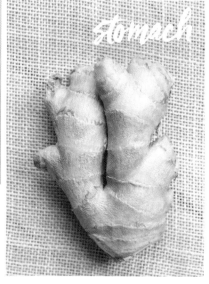

stomach

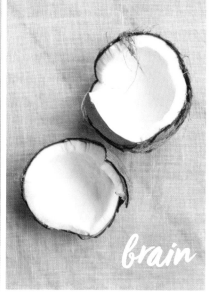

brain

doctrine of signatures

This philosophy dates back to the sixteenth century, when it was believed that foods and herbs resembled the element of the body they were meant to heal or bring wellness to. Although there is no scientific basis for the Doctrine of Signatures, it's nonetheless true that some fruit and vegetables out there resemble the part of the body they are good for, which makes for a fun little exercise. For example, celery is good for bone health and resembles bones; tomatoes are good for heart health and the inside of a tomato looks like the chambers of a heart. This practice also promotes mindful, intuitive eating practices. This is a simple way to think about how to nourish ourself intentionally.

Check out this photographic chart with descriptions of the parts of our body that benefit from each food. Give this ritual a whirl by selecting the food that is meant to nourish a part of your body that needs a little extra TLC.

women's gathering: play to learn

Over the years, I've found that women's groups provide a safe space for us ladies. Here we can feel secure in opening up and sharing our vulnerabilities and we can find support and opportunities for love and growth. I can't stress this enough:

Making the time to be with our girlfriends is vitally important. It deprograms us from the cultural mentality that teaches us we need to compete and win and, instead, teaches us to simply be and to play. We can use our voice, and share our insights and visions to empower both ourself and others. We can experience a renewed feminism through making time and space for enriching experiences that allow us to connect and go further together, to move beyond boundaries, and to design a more sustainable inner and outer world. Perhaps best of all, we can inspire one another to always go forward and to be strong.

In addition to supporting one another's goals and intentions, these gatherings allow us a regular opportunity to foster deep, supportive relationships with other women. They offer the chance to play with our friends, to support them when things are difficult, to celebrate their successes, and to support one another's intentions. These gatherings create a long-term, effective, and sustainable sense of psychological safety and collaborative intelligence between us and our girlfriends.

Here are some of my favorite gathering themes, although you should also feel free to get creative and come up with your own.

New Moon Gatherings

The new moon is associated with new beginnings, so these gatherings generally entail intention-setting, but can also include everything from food and cocktails to educational opportunities through guest lecturers, and so on. I am a big fan of bringing women together, whatever the occasion may be, but new moons are a particularly powerful time to do so.

Organizing Parties

Is there a cause that you feel especially passionate about? Bringing a group together around that cause is a good way to dialogue about the issue, set objectives, and determine strategies and tactics to make a difference. It feels great to champion a cause with a group of your fellow concerned citizens who share common goals and want to create change in the world.

Book Club

It is so much fun to dive in and discuss a book with other women. It's enlightening to hear how others analyze the same book from their unique perspective. While discussing the book, there is also the opportunity to share personal anecdotes, reflect, and learn about the triumph and struggles of others, while also learning more about yourself in the process.

Slow Beauty Gatherings

Create a support group around your Slow Beauty practice. Do some of the exercises in this book together, make some of the recipes, and even perform the movement exercises together. Share your own recipes and rituals. Have a Slow Beauty workshop to map it all out.

HOW TO DO IT

(1) Determine what type of group you would like to start: New Moon gathering, Slow Beauty practice group, book club, organizing party, or any other theme that excites you. The main point here is to carve out and make a commitment to this time spent together.

(2) Decide whether you want to make this an intimate type of group or something more social. I find that seven to eight women is a good number for book clubs, to facilitate a robust discussion where everyone has an opportunity to contribute. For New Moon gatherings, organizing parties, or Slow Beauty practice groups, seven to eight women is a great number for an intimate vibe; fifteen to eighteen is ideal for sharing, idea generation, and socializing. You may want to invite the same guests to participate in the group every time or you may prefer a rotating roster. I have found that larger gatherings tend to have a core group of women who attend each gathering, and

others who come from time to time. There is no right or wrong way to do it.

(3) Decide where you would like to host your gathering. I find that hosting at home is comfortable and cozy, but hosting outside of the home to have new experiences, explore, and mix it up can be nice, too.

(4) Offering food is always a good idea. Potlucks are a great option, and a nice opportunity for sharing.

(5) I find two hours is generally a good amount of time for the larger groups as these are often more structured affairs with a guest speaker or a specific objective. For intimate groups, I usually forgo a time limit and let the gathering unfold and progress organically.

(6) Monthly meetings work well for both book clubs and New Moon groups. For organizing parties, set the gatherings based on your group's objective and the urgency of the issue at hand. For Slow Beauty practice gatherings, weekly, biweekly, or monthly are all viable options.

(7) If you are gathering with an intimate group, pick your next meeting date based on everyone's schedules before the end of each gathering. You may also want to consider rotating from house to house. For larger groups, announce the next date at the end of your gathering, then follow up with an invite.

classes and services

Although Slow Beauty is meant to be self-sufficient and practiced in the comfort of our own homes and time frames, it is always fun to try some of the unique classes and services that are up for offer within our communities. Experiment with different classes and services outside of your normal routine to inspire and stimulate your mind, body, and soul. It's also a great opportunity to remove ourself from our comfort zone. (In other words, if you already practice yoga regularly, give something else on this list a whirl. You never know! You may just find something you love.) Here are some ideas to get you started.

- Dance classes
- Lectures
- Live music
- Meditation classes
- Museums
- Salon visits
- Shirodhara (Ayurvedic treatment)
- Sound baths
- Spa treatments
- Strength-training

poetics: speak to your soul

As with philosophy, we have also lost touch with the great poems and poets. It's a shame, too, because poetry elevates, renews, and transforms us by helping us transcend the mundane. This Poetics ritual is designed to engage us with the beauty of poetry and to help us live a more poetic life by immersing us in poems that inspire and uplift on a seasonal basis.

The role of the poet is to tend the soul of the world. Poets are interpreters of feelings. They give shape to invisible feelings unspoken, and a voice to the silent language alive in the space between the words. Poets highlight the nuances in the movements of the language of the body and in the fits and starts of human communication. Poetry is self-healing; it cleanses our soul. Poets are givers, they are lovers. Walt Whitman said that the poem is a temple within which we can truly feel our feelings. Be a poet.

I recommend reading one poem daily. This might look any number of different ways. You may read the same poem daily for a week, a month, or a year. You may read a new, different poem each day. You can—and should!—read poetry any way you wish. Just read it. Poetry speaks directly to and nourishes the soul, touching it with light and healing it. Poems have the ability to awaken that which has been asleep or numbed. Sometimes a poem might affect you so profoundly as to open up something inside of you and deliver you to your soul.

Here you will find some recommendations for poems and poets to get you started. You can find most of these poems on poets.org—and, not only that, the site is also a great place to do some discovery on your own. If a poem either on this list or from any other source speaks to you, I recommend writing it in the Notes pages at the end of this book for your reference, to add to your Slow Beauty practice.

These poems are organized by season, although they may be read at any time throughout the year. Read them to yourself, read them aloud, sing them, whatever feels right to you!

I found God in myself and I loved her. I loved her fiercely.

—NTOZAKE SHANGE

Winter

"I Will Keep Broken Things" by Alice Walker

"Be Nobody's Darling" by Alice Walker

"Expect Nothing" by Alice Walker

"Still I Rise" by Maya Angelou

"A Myth of Devotion" by Louise Gluck

"Ode to My Socks" by Pablo Neruda

Spring

"End of Winter" by Louise Gluck

"Written in March" by William Wordsworth

"A Blessing" by James Wright

"The Awakening" by Rumi

Summer

"Midsummer" by Louise Gluck

"Out Here" by Ursula K. Le Guin

"Artistic Statement" by Denise Duhamel

"The Subject Tonight Is Love" by Hafiz

Fall

"I Wandered Lonely as a Cloud"
    by William Wordsworth

"Learning the Name" by Ursula K. Le Guin

"Sonnet VII (O Solitude! If I Must with Thee
    Dwell)" by John Keats

And if you're looking for poems based on a specific theme or topic, here are some more suggestions:

DAILY LIFE: Pablo Neruda

ECSTASY: Hafiz

FREEDOM AND INDIVIDUALITY: Alice Walker

IDENTITY: Maya Angelou

INTROVERSION: Mary Oliver

LOSS AND ISOLATION: Louise Gluck

NATURE AND FANTASY: Ursula K. Le Guin

NATURE AND MAN: William Wordsworth

PASSION: Rumi

ROMANCE: John Keats

SEPARATION: James Wright

WIT: Denise Duhamel

self-symposium: be a great mind

Our quest with this ritual is to harness our thought process until it becomes second nature. We also aim to create space and illuminate the answers, new ideas, and concepts present inside of us that are being muddled and weighed down by the incessant chatter of a distracted, anxious, and stressed-out mind. The dialogue we'll create through this ritual should be a stimulating, energizing sort of spiritual warfare. The purpose is to deepen, strengthen, and bring light to the thoughts floating in our mind. It is to understand which thoughts to just let go of and which thoughts to build upon. This is the art of virtuous thinking and clarity of mind.

This ritual is inspired by the famous ancient Greek symposiums and, specifically, Plato's philosophical text *Symposium*, wherein philosophers at a dinner party have a discourse about the concept of love, its nature, and its purpose. In the course of this conversation, ancient prophetess Diotima explains that she considers the greatest form of love between two people to be chiefly educational and philosophical in nature. And so it is with the self. We have the opportunity to elevate the conversations we have with *ourself*, wherein our inner dialogue becomes generative, creative, fluid, self-possessed, and positive.

We can take the sage advice of Eleanor Roosevelt and apply it to our conversations with ourself as well. As she put it, "Great minds discuss ideas, average minds discuss events, small minds discuss people." We are what we think, so why not form habits around productive thinking processes and practice the virtue of a strong and discerning mind?

We should all question our assumptions and the stories we tell ourself. So many of our assumptions are based on old, outdated thought patterns that we learned in and carried forth from childhood. A meditation practice can definitely help hone our thought patterns in this way. Meditation shows us how thoughts simply come and go. It helps us to create space between our thoughts and our self and puts us in the position of objective observer. This positioning gives us a bird's-eye view of a situation, and seeing the bigger picture helps us to be less reactive. This, in turn, improves the health of our central nervous system, not to mention our overall health and well-being.

All too often, we seek answers from outside sources that may or may not resonate with us or be aligned with who we are. Through this exercise, we will learn how to begin to have a dialogue with ourself in a Socratic way. We will begin by asking ourself questions. This is essentially a meeting of our own mind and a way of getting in touch with different aspects of ourself. It allows us to be in conversation with our higher self, God, nature, the infinite, or whatever you want to call "it."

We want to facilitate a self-reflexive dialogue that will help elevate our internal conversations. This is important because our thoughts are malleable things that appear in our mind. They come and go. Some thoughts come in and quickly fade away; others, we grasp on to, forging an attachment to and further shaping them. We build on these thoughts and give them texture, volume, weight, longitude, and latitude. We can build on such thoughts in a variety of ways. Sometimes this includes unconsciously doing so in negative ways that can turn toxic and affect not only our mind, but also have a powerful physical and emotional impact. Know this: You are fully in charge of how you develop and build out those thoughts that pop into your head.

Quite often we are challenged externally. Something happens outside of us—someone says something that pushes our buttons or we say or do something that doesn't make us feel good afterward—and resulting thoughts pop in and start to spiral out of control. And that's not even to mention what happens internally. We have varying viewpoints inside of us. Because of this, we often avoid making decisions altogether because we are so internally fragmented about where our best interests lie. So, we suffer in indecision. Or we constantly have thousands of thoughts racing through our mind, many of which are wreaking havoc on our central nervous system by causing a heightened state of anxiety and stress. The purpose of this ritual is to stop the spiraling and indecision and, over time, to become a master of our own mind. I know—very aspirational. But it's a good and worthy pursuit.

A few things to keep in mind before we get started: With this self-symposium, there are no winners or losers because it isn't a competition; it is a process through which a consensus and a feeling of satisfaction are attained. The objective is to help you reach an internal consensus about the truth—your truth. In the course of this, some of our virtues are called into play—we must be patient, thoughtful, tolerant, and compassionate with ourself as we embark upon this quest for our inner truth. It is a rational discourse to shed light on and illuminate an answer to a question that you have been mentally grappling with. Perhaps you're thinking, "But I have no questions to answer." Often, we don't even realize those questions that dwell inside of us. It isn't until we slow down for a long enough period for them to pop into our mind that they become apparent. With that in mind, when performed on a regular basis, this ritual can help us connect with our questions and answers on a more frequent basis, thus keeping our mind more regulated. Remember, this is not a brainstorming session, but a methodical investigation inspired by the Socratic method of using questioning as a means of energized critical thinking and illuminating new ideas to help alleviate the issues and pains in our life.

Ready to get started? You can do this ritual first thing in the morning to start your day with a clear head, to cleanse your mind before bed in the evening for a more restful night's sleep, or at the first sign of a thought that has become rebellious. You will need a pen, and a journal—I would recommend designating a self-symposium journal that you reserve specifically for this exercise. You'll also find some space at the end of this book to use for your very first self-symposium. Feel free to enjoy a glass of organic wine as you complete this ritual (after all, wine was always served at these symposiums), and reap the age-defying benefits of resveratrol as you clear your mind.

Now that you're ready to roll, there are two approaches to this art of thinking. Choose whichever works best for you and, of course, you may find that different strategies serve you in different scenarios.

① Why? So?

Start with a statement like "I hate my job" and then continue down the page asking and responding to the questions "Why?" and "So?" Continue writing for as long as it takes to empty your brain and thoroughly answer the questions. When you've finished, read back through your musings, highlighting any illuminations and/or breakthroughs that resonate with you. Find those revelations that are virtuous and beautiful and true to you, then build upon and develop them further, nurturing the most gorgeous, productive, feel-good thoughts in your head and leaving the rest on your paper.

② The Question

Start with a question like "What does beauty mean to me?" Answer that question with brief, simple, unemotional statements written in first person (e.g., "I believe beauty is . . ."). Write down all of the responses that come to mind without editing—that will come later. Once you've compiled your answers, expand on each of those answers with another question specific to the answer. Continue with this process until you've broken through and developed your thought into a dynamic composition worthy of contemplation. Thoughts that bring you down, upset you, or induce anxiety or stress belong in the garbage dump, not the Museum of Modern Art.

bibliotherapy

Bibliotherapy is a unique form of therapy wherein we identify something we need and then read a prescription of books as a form of therapy to help resolve the issue at hand. Connecting with characters and information directly related to our current life experience reaches us in ways other forms of therapy do not. Books also provide an opportunity for psychological safety. We are free to explore and experience our breadth of emotions and thoughts without external pressures, biases, opinions, or interruptions. Bibliotheraphy is about nourishing ourself and reading itself helps us to slow down and reduce stress.

As long-form reading is becoming less and less common, it's all too easy to forget the multisensory benefits of holding a book in our hands and turning the pages. Books are tactile and they have a smell that e-books simply do not. Not to mention the fact that reading an actual book is way more forgiving on our eyes.

Following are some categorized reading sets that promote self-actualization. Curl up and get cozy as you dive in and let go!

Goodness

If you desire kindness and want to delve deeper into the nuances of love, these books will give you the keys you need for access.

Quiet by Susan Cain

The Power of Kindness by Piero Ferrucci

The Art of Loving by Erich Fromm

In Praise of Slowness by Carl Honore

Inner Life

The books in this set will help you begin the process of getting in touch with your inner world.

The House of Fulfillment by L. Adams Beck

The Secret Language of Tarot by Wald Amberstone and Ruth Ann Amberstone

Inner Work by Robert A. Johnson

The Invisible Partners by John A. Sanford

The Heroine's Journey by Maureen Murdock

Wild-Natured Woman

Are you a wild woman? Do you often feel like you are going against the grain? This set will support you in connecting more with your wild, feminine nature, and setting it free. You will be moved to express your wildness out in the world in positive, healthy ways.

Women Who Run with the Wolves by Clarissa Pinkola Estés

The Snow Child by Eowyn Ivey

Awakening the Heroes Within by Carol Pearson

Daughters of Saturn by Patricia Reis

Sacred Pleasure by Riane Eisler

Return to Nature

Do you long to be immersed in nature? Have a closer connection and relationship with nature as *the* infinite, eternal source of inspiration and innovation? Start here.

Biomimicry by Janine M. Benyus

Silent Spring by Rachel Carson

Staying Healthy with the Seasons by
    Elson M. Haas

Last Child in the Woods by Richard Louv

Earthing by Clinton Ober, Stephen T. Sinatra,
    and Martin Zucker

Passionate Self

Do you long to be in deep communication with yourself? Warm, intimate, and deeply loving, this set will spark the fire of passionate conversation with yourself.

Anam Cara by John O'Donohue

Upstream by Mary Oliver

*Reflections on the Art of Living: A Joseph
    Campbell Companion* selected and edited by
    Diane K. Osbon

Bend Your Mind

Are you fascinated by the inner workings of the mind? Are you someone who thinks differently? This set will excite your brain.

Neurodiversity by Thomas Armstrong

A Whole New Mind by Daniel H. Pink

Word Encounters

Are you moved to write? Do you long for the creative life? These books will bring you inside the creative process of a writer, a thinker, and a dancer, *and* introduce you to some characters who were transformed by artistic expression. Your creative work matters. We need you to create.

Meditations by Marcus Aurelius

The Writing Life by Annie Dillard

Bird by Bird by Anne Lamott

Balzac and the Little Chinese Seamstress
    by Dai Sijie

The Creative Habit by Twyla Tharp

social good

What is more beautiful than helping others? Here are some ways to get out there and make the world beautiful, just like you. And, in the process of doing good, you'll feel better and more beautiful, too. It's a gorgeous cycle! Giving back not only helps the world, but it also helps us by releasing the feel-good hormone oxytocin, which elevates our mood. The knowledge that we are making a difference in the world also provides us with a sense of purpose and meaning. In fact, a Harvard School of Public Health study revealed that people who volunteer spend less time in hospitals. So, volunteering might also just save your life!

Make an impact locally in your community or globally. Purchase brands that give back so you are using products you love *and* doing something great for the planet at the same time. On a day-to-day basis, be more than just a consumer—be a citizen of the world.

Here are some resources to help connect you with volunteer opportunities, both in your neighborhood and globally.

Apps
Deed
Elev8society

Websites
Crowdrise.com
Dosomething.org
Volunteermatch.org

Animal Rights
Gentlebarn.org
Mercyforanimals.org
Peta.org

Environmental
Greenpeace.org
Sierraclub.org
Slowfood.com

Health Advocacy
Plannedparenthood.org
Policywell.org

Literacy and Education
Jstart.org
Roomtoread.org
Ymadvocacy.org

Women's Rights
Equalitynow.org
Theelders.org
Thestrongmovement.com
Womensmarch.com

emotion blending

Don't believe the hype that emotions are either good or bad. They're also not trendy. Emotions are the classical, infinitely everlasting notes of the song of your life. We speak so much about diversity and its importance, but somehow we relegate diversity to the tone of our skin, our cultural heritage, and our socioeconomic status. What of the diversity of our emotional relationship with the world? There are both intellectual and emotional ways to relate to the world, but we are so judgmental about the range of emotions we are allowed to express. There are the good emotions we are allowed and even pushed to reveal, such as enthusiasm, happiness, and gratitude. And the others, well, those are relegated to some distant, dusty corner deep within and buried under layers of other unacceptable emotions, where they wait, festering, and may explode at any moment because we have no forum through which to process them.

Emotions are the elixir, the sap that oozes from us when we've been tapped. So many of our emotions are so fresh and new and different, but we stop them from flowing, because they don't belong in the clique of emotions that have been sanctioned by society as acceptable. How ridiculous is this?!

We become alive when we feel and when we aren't afraid of the feelings we are feeling. Unfortunately, we have this cultural code of a limited range of emotions we are allowed to feel and share with others. In reality, emotions are like a symphony. Each emotion is an instrument, and the notes played from the instrument are the layers of the emotions.

We can also think of emotions as colors, as social psychologist William McDougall noted in 1921 when he identified a parallel between colors and emotions. Within each color is a range of shadings depicting the complexity of an emotion. Although our experience of emotions is complex, our language around them is usually one-dimensional. We are disconnected from the hue, texture, breadth, and depth each emotion contains. Which brings me to Robert Plutchik, who in 1958 identified eight basic emotions that are polar opposites: joy versus sorrow, anger versus fear, acceptance versus disgust, and surprise versus expectancy. In the 1980s, Plutchik created a way to classify emotions in a model he called the Wheel of Emotions.* This wheel combines his list of polar opposite emotion sets with McDougall's concept of emotional shading. This wheel, which can be easily found online, gives us a visual for what is otherwise an internal state that is difficult to explain. According to the wheel, in the same way that two primary colors are mixed together to create a third color, basic emotions can be blended together to create new emotions. For example, according to the wheel, when serenity and interest are blended together, they create optimism. This is important to acknowledge because often we experience a blend of

*Robert Plutchik, "The Nature of Emotions," *American Scientist* 89.

emotions that is difficult to articulate because they are so layered, and we've never learned the layered language of emotions.

Using Plutchik's wheel, we are going to create emotional blends. Say, you want to feel more optimistic. Your blend will require you to feel serenity and interest to get to the emotion of optimism. What makes you feel serene? Is it taking a walk in nature? Reading a book? And what sparks your interest? Speaking to a good friend about a topic that interests you? Or attending a class about a topic that's new to you? Combine those external stimuli that make you feel serene and interested to mix yourself up some optimism.

As you play with this wheel, make sure you don't shy away from the emotions that aren't so popular, such as the annoyance and boredom that blend together to create contempt. I know, who would want to feel those emotions on purpose? Well, you aren't always in control of what triggers these emotions, so if you experiment with them in a more "controlled environment," it will be easier for you to understand and deal with contempt when it rises up out of nowhere. Having already blended contempt, you will know that underlying it is a layer of boredom and annoyance, and that you have the power to identify and shift your focus to another emotional blend.

broken teacup ritual

As you wake up to the ways in which you have been neglecting yourself, this ritual will be very helpful. Remember the Japanese practice of kintsigu? There is a psychological concept of self-therapy that expresses this same idea. A largely unknown Polish psychoanalyst and psychologist, Kazimierz Dabrowski, who was prolific between 1929 and 1981, was friends with Abraham Maslow, among other noted psychologists. Dabrowski developed the Theory of Positive Disintegration. Like kintsigu, this theory is a paradox. Dabrowski saw value in "falling apart" and beauty in allowing ourself and our fixed perspectives to "disintegrate" for growth to occur. We don't need to hold it together all of the time. There are moments when we may need to just fall apart. In fact, this is *necessary* to grow and become a better version of ourself, according to Dabrowski.

We live in a society where the pursuit of perfection and excellence is paramount, and when we do have moments of despair or feel out of control, we experience feelings of guilt and shame. We don't expose our vulnerabilities because it challenges society's norm of perfectionism and the myopic pursuit of excellence. Of course we want to be the best version of ourself; however, along the way it is necessary to give ourself permission to enact radical inclusivity and hold with compassion those aspects of ourself that are not considered beautiful by today's standards. This self-therapy ritual is

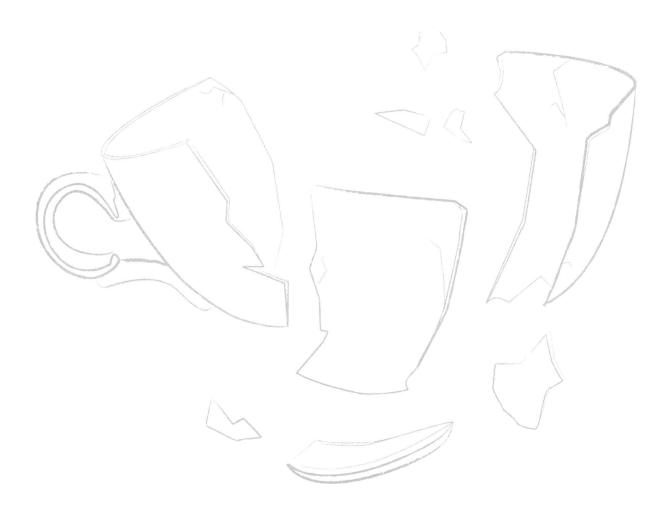

an opportunity to "fall apart" and put ourself back together again with a realignment of values, based on our inner beliefs, and a renewed connection to our individual essence. The outcome is a new pathway toward a higher level of intrapersonal development and knowing.

Begin this ritual by gazing upon the image of the broken teacup above. Title the image an event or experience in your life where you felt as if you "fell apart." In the spaces or cracks between the pieces, write what you learned from that experience that caused you to fall apart, and how it changed you. These are your "golden threads," the light you have gleaned from a challenging experience. This is how you put yourself back together after having fallen apart.

your personal crest

In the Middle Ages, families often represented their values and status in the world with a personal crest, or a shield that contained symbols relating to their family tradition and history. An image of a crown might be used to convey that they were part of the royal family; a dog might serve as a symbol of loyalty and friendship; and even the colors selected for the shield often had a specific meaning and intention. As we make our own personal crests in this ritual, we will have the opportunity to slow down and identify what values are the most important to us and define us most.

(1) Title the crest in the space with your name. Alternatively, feel free to use a name you've always wished you'd been called, or a nickname that you prefer. Or it could be a word that motivates and inspires you, such as *victory*. Whatever you want. This is your coat of arms.

(2) Choose your color palette for the background and in the drawings.

(3) Choose a terrain, such as the ocean, mountain, forest, or a desert, and draw it at the bottom of the shield.

(4) Choose an animal that best describes who you are (if you need some help, check out the Animal Totem section on page 191). This might be a single animal or an animal composite; for example, the body of a lion, eyes of a hawk, and feet of a rooster. Draw or collage the animal in the center of the crest on top of the terrain.

(5) Embellish the rest of your crest with other symbols that are meaningful to you, such as flowers, stars, other animals, books, or whatever feels right. Your imagination is the limit!

Once you've completed your personal crest, write about why you chose to include what you included. Write down everything that comes to mind: What does the color mean to you? The animal? Now write about how you make this crest central to your daily life. How will you use the crest? Will it be a form of protection? Inspiration? Aspiration? How often will you renew your crest?

role playing

Most of us are juggling so many roles. Way more than we consciously realize on a moment-to-moment basis. For example, I am a mother, wife, daughter, founder, writer, sister, and friend. These are the roles I mostly embody. In the past and from time to time, I play other roles as well, but those I just listed are the ones I occupy for the majority of my time. Pause for a moment and list all of the roles that pertain to you.

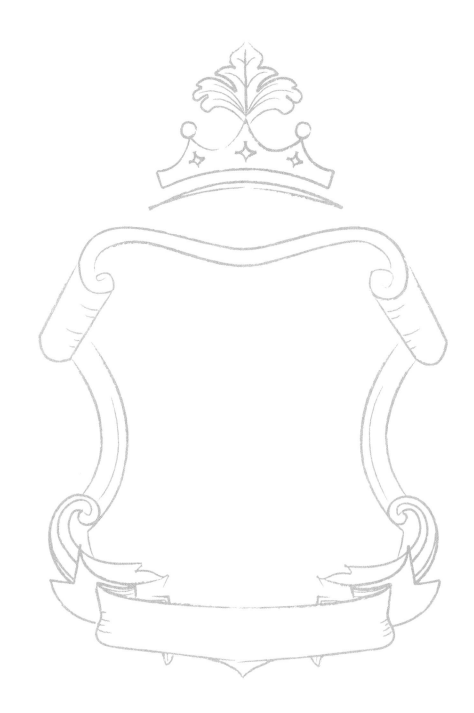

Choose your colors and create your personal coat of arms.

Now that you have your list of roles, rank them in the order of the time you spend in that role. Are there roles on the list that you need or want to give more shape, meaning, or texture? If so, raise those roles up to a higher ranking. Remove any roles that are no longer serving you or in your best interests.

Now, one by one, remove each role. Write down the roles you would like to play. Perhaps you are a feminist or an activist at heart, but that role either receded to the background or was never realized because you became occupied being a working mother.

Finally, ask your friends and family members what they perceive as your major roles. This will give you yet another perspective.

Now that you have all of this information, it's time to get to work. Reanimate those roles that are meaningful to you and might have been lost, while retiring the ones that no longer serve you. Allow yourself to become the person you want to be, to play the role or roles you want to play.

growing young

In the Philosophy section, we looked at the twenty-seven neotenous traits as identified by Montagu, plus one additional trait of understanding. Perhaps you've noted that there are subtle opportunities strewn throughout this book to experience these traits. Here's one more.

This ritual is designed to help you to connect with the idea of growing young. Each one of these traits (see page 25 for a refresher) shapes a path to health, and paves the way to true beauty—understanding what your needs are, identifying which of these attributes you need to nourish more, igniting more of them into your life, and really defining for yourself how to express these attributes in your life, in your way, at your pace, in your terms. How can you thread them together in such a way that you can create a beautiful tapestry of your uniqueness?

Meditate on these traits at least weekly and jot down some ideas that come to mind in terms of how you can experience them. Here's the thing: You *know* what you need, you just need to slow down long enough for the answer to expose itself to you so that you can isolate that trait as something that will benefit your health, well-being, and beauty. Make it like a meal plan, and nourish yourself with joy for breakfast, dance for lunch, and optimism for dinner. Or declare a monodiet of one of the traits, such as laughter, and do a laughter cleanse, which requires no more than just starting to laugh. It will feel forced at first and then, suddenly, it will turn into real, authentic laughter.

Ingest, digest, integrate, and continue doing so until you really expand these traits to the point where they are so ingrained in you that they become infectious, and you actually light them up in others.

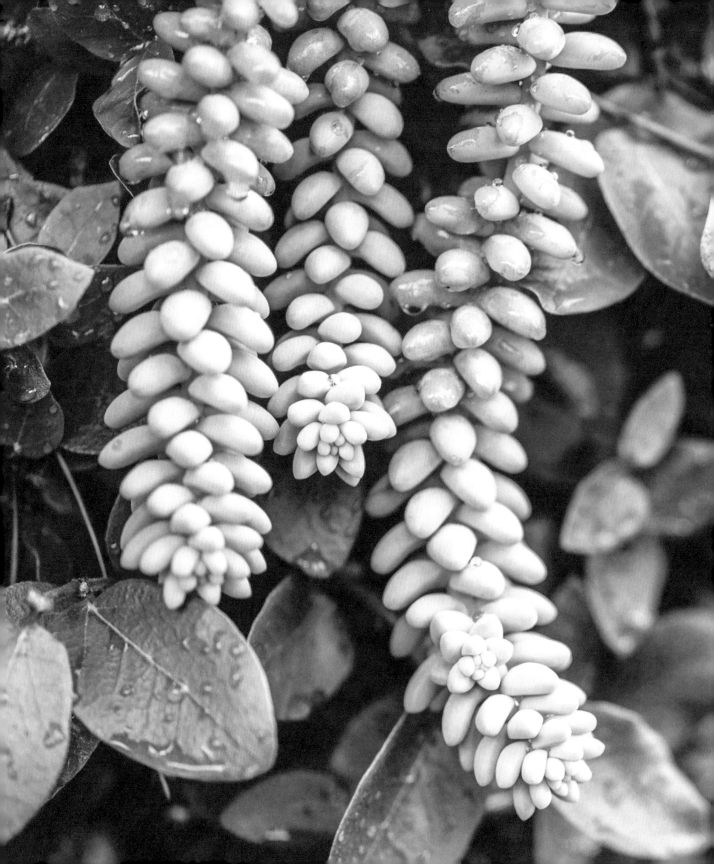

Part Three:

RECIPES

*As you sow
so shall you reap.*

—BIBLE, GALATIANS VI

SOME OF THE RECIPES WE ARE ABOUT TO DELVE INTO ARE TRADITIONAL IN THE sense that they are actual food recipes. You'll also find recipes for movement, meditation, and DIY body care products. The commonality between all of these recipes is that, as with rituals, these recipes are intentional and require our presence of mind, body, and spirit, both in making and in experiencing them. They focus us in the now and place us in a meditative or mindful state. Also like rituals, these recipes are a tool for harnessing our otherwise scattered trove of energy.

They offer us yet another way to transform a pressured life into a precious life. As we make and experience these recipes—selecting organic ingredients whenever possible—we are seizing an opportunity to slow down, to savor the moment and the silence. We simplify. In this process, we can take some inspiration from natural asceticism, becoming more mindful about what and how we consume, as well as of our relationship with consumerism. Asceticism has been criticized for its extremity, and rightly so. To be clear, in the context of Slow Beauty, we'll think of asceticism as consuming the right things in moderation.

The objective of the recipes you'll find in this chapter is to create a state of calm and uplifted wholeness. They will help us decrease stress, anxiety, and worry. They will balance the central nervous system so that we can naturally experience more expansive states of consciousness. It is through these expanded states of consciousness that we can cultivate and maintain an ongoing sense of joy—the type of joy that is like a flame that never goes out, even if it is dimmer at some points than others. Regardless of its brightness, the quality of that glowing light is always warming, calming, and uplifting; its brightness simply varies depending upon our internal season.

These recipes give our central nervous system a break, which is crucial because it is in doing this that we get to what author Peter Russell calls "the quieter underlying levels of thinking" in his book *From Science to God*. It is in this withdrawal from the craziness of day-to-day doing that we are given the opportunity to tap into the expansiveness of consciousness itself. With this comes renewal and, in turn, we are able to create anew. When our central nervous system is pacified, we are open to experience the more expansive aspects of consciousness, both internally and externally.

the slow beauty of consciousness

I know, I know. There is a lot of talk about consciousness these days: higher consciousness, expanded consciousness, raising consciousness. This is probably because, on some level, we all understand that it's time for a change. And to really change things, to make the world a better place, requires a major shift in consciousness for the simple reason that the way we have been approaching things is not working. And our current approaches aren't working, mostly because we are not *in consciousness* so much of the time. We are somewhere else—in the past, in the future, in physical pain, in mental pain, in emotional pain. Because of these other things, our experience of consciousness is extremely limited and narrow. We can break out of this by focusing on the positive, sharing the light, studying healthy people, and gaining an understanding of what makes us as individuals healthy.

But what does consciousness have to do with Slow Beauty? Everything. Developing a Slow Beauty practice will help you raise your consciousness. With this, your entire life experience is more peaceful and magical. The entire point of having a Slow Beauty practice is to feel the joy; it is

through being in the highest state of consciousness that we experience joy and bliss. To achieve these higher states, we have to clear away all of the distractions that occupy us in body and in mind. This includes such things as overtaxing the digestive system by eating poorly, shallow breathing, and restricted movement.

Consciousness is the new frontier. But what is it? Where is it? Consciousness is something that can't be directly described, so it is often described in metaphor. Most of the time the experience of consciousness cannot be described at all. To describe it would require an entirely new language. We speak the language of the waking state of consciousness. There are many other states. Mystics and seekers have attempted to explain their unique experience of consciousness for ages.

Consciousness is found both inside and outside ourself. It is something we can access when our central nervous system is calm. It is a source of awareness—always present, infinite, and eternal. It is always there for us; we only need to unplug from the chaos and distractions of the world and plug into consciousness instead. When we raise our consciousness, we lighten the load of our per-

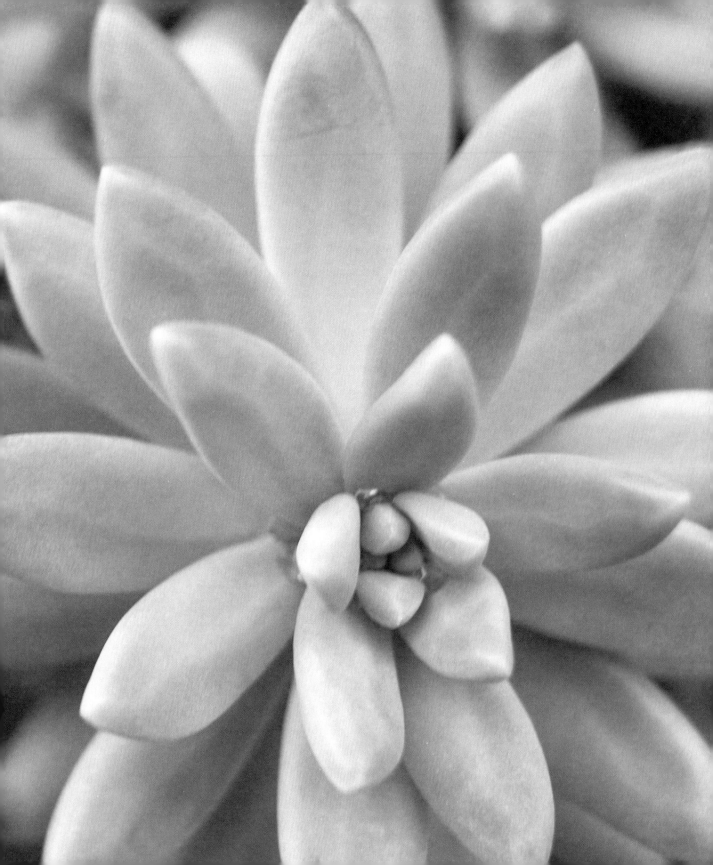

sonal burdens until we reach the point where we can rise above those burdens altogether.

For many, like myself, this attainment of greater consciousness is a mission. I spend a lot of time reading about and researching consciousness because the subject fascinates me, and I'm fully committed to expanding my own consciousness. It isn't always an easy process, and I absolutely stumble along the way, but patiently I forge ahead, identifying and facing my obstacles, being honest about my limitations and taking the time to unravel those things that catch me and trip me up, always assuring myself that I'll have the opportunity to do it better the next time around. Because that thing that trips us up will come around again, until we make peace with it.

STATES OF CONSCIOUSNESS

In his book *From Science to God,* Peter Russell explains consciousness as a faculty that is always present, everywhere, and in everything. As part of everything, we are forms of consciousness. Our central nervous system, our organs, and our thoughts amplify consciousness. When we balance and purify these things, our experience of consciousness will be that much more profound, robust, and expansive. Higher levels of consciousness allow us to energetically vibrate in a way that allows us to fluidly and easily access the twenty-seven growing young needs. As a result of this, our life will feel and be fuller, more peaceful, and more enjoyable than ever before. The following is a list defining some of the different states of consciousness.

(1) **WAKING:** what you do each day, your struggles, emotions, dramas, etc.

(2) **DREAMING:** how you process the waking life, problem-solving, unconscious fantasies, etc.

(3) **DEEP SLEEPING:** the state in which your body and mind rest completely; when we are in this state, there is no visual aspect of dreaming.

(4) **IN BETWEEN:** this state exists between waking and deep sleeping, and involves feelings of deep relaxation, bliss, and joy that extend into the waking state when we reenter it. It is accessible when we intentionally utilize such consciousness tools as Yoga Nidra (see page 183) or Transcendental Meditation.

consciousness and the central nervous system

It is only through slowing down that we will be able to comprehend the nuances of the states of consciousness. The central nervous system is like our own personal central intelligence or ground control. If our central nervous system is disorganized, disillusioned, anxious, overworked, or highly stressed, then the state of consciousness we experience will be dull and lackluster. Nourish the system, feed the system, care for the system in deep and meaningful ways, and then the barriers and blockages are removed so we can access the higher states of consciousness. These higher states have been described as feelings of joy and bliss. We use meditation and other techniques to tap into these experiences. Imagine if we are able to plug into consciousness and bring it into our waking state! I'm here to tell you that we can through the philosophies, rituals, and recipes in this book. And the more we do it, the more seamless this process becomes. It is as if we are bringing things back from our trip to consciousness and weaving them into our waking state.

The central nervous system contains the sympathetic and parasympathetic pathways that control our response to danger and regulation of bodily functions. These include hormone release, movement of food through the stomach and intestines, and the sensations from and muscular control of all internal organs.

The sympathetic nervous system—often referred to as "fight or flight"—is the part of the central nervous system that prepares us for intense activity. The parasympathetic nervous system does the opposite; it helps us rest and digest, relaxes the body, and often slows down high levels of energy. The more we calm the sympathetic nervous system and activate the parasympathetic nervous system, the easier it will be to tap into our consciousness. It is the sympathetic part of the nervous system that is being challenged by today's fast world. We are too tense, too sped up. We need to use the tools and techniques available to us to help our parasympathetic nervous system engage. It is through this that we will achieve a state of calm, reduce our heart rate, and relax our muscles—all of those things that help us to heal, restore, renew, and come back to ourself. This is, in large part, the intent behind the recipes you'll find in this section of the book—to assist in cultivating an optimally functioning central nervous system.

CREATE A HOUSE OF FULFILLMENT

As you move through the recipes in this chapter, I encourage you to keep in mind the idea of *shalom bayit*. This is a Jewish concept that means "peace in the home" or "peace between husband and wife." I love this concept as a metaphor for the relationship of a fully integrated self. Since our body is the home in which we reside, it is through the body that we can cultivate a self that is whole and in balance. To attain this peaceful home for ourself, we must have the courage to slow down and reflect on what is working for us and what is not. From there, the rest is simple. Keep doing what works, identify what isn't, and do the work to remove the barriers to your expansion.

seasons come and seasons go

I've categorized the recipes in this section by season, but with one little twist: I'm asking you to think of seasons as a state of being, feeling, and thinking, rather than as a time of the year. Remember, Slow Beauty has everything to do with tapping into your own internal rhythms, and these may or may not correspond with the time of year the calendar shows us. These internal seasons will relate to the qualities of the external seasons to which we are accustomed. We have our unique cycles, and phases of life. Sometimes, we are in a winterlike season of melancholy; other times, we are in a season of extreme expressiveness, like spring.

To honor ourself, it is so important that we identify the season we are in and abide by it.

If this all sounds a bit esoteric, don't fret! This chapter will help you identify the qualities each season expresses, so that you can easily tap into and harness it when appropriate. Living in this intentional and connected way helps us to internalize the cycles of life and our place in it at any given moment. In doing this, we begin to understand that change is inevitable, important, and necessary for continual growth to occur. It also reminds us that phases are temporal and temporary, which opens us up to a healthier, more open-

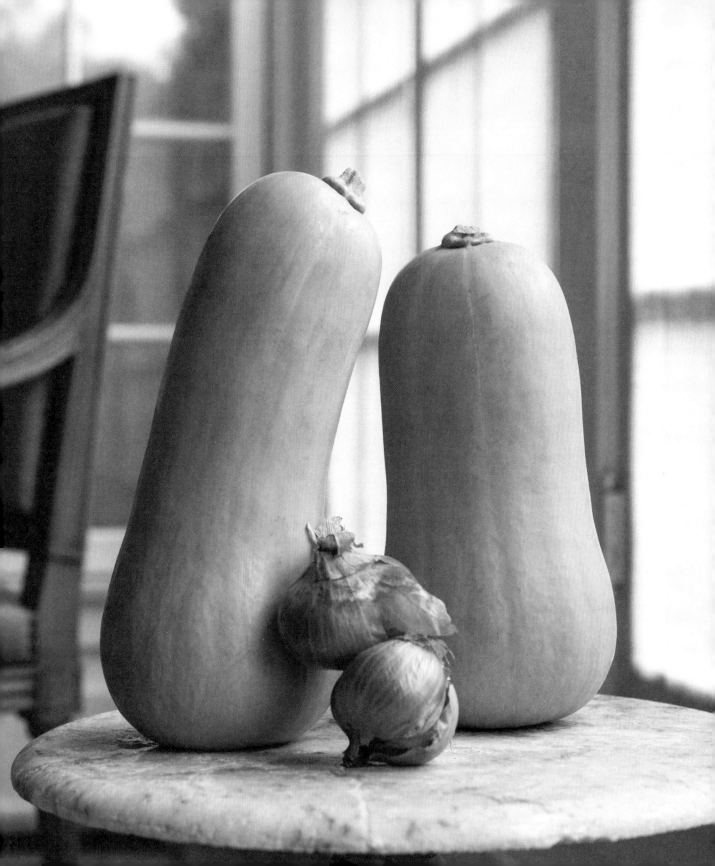

minded "this too shall pass" mentality. It frees us from being stuck or sticky. We can stop grasping onto emotions, attempting to cling to them so that they stick around. After all, what comes up must come down, and what is down always has the ability to go up again. It is gravitational law.

These seasonal attributes are inspired by the practice of Chinese medicine, which focuses on elements, and the Indian practice of Ayurveda, which focuses on our individual body constitution. Both are seasonal-based practices of well-being and address the balances and imbalances each season contains, as well as the qualities and essence of each season. Tuning into these cycles helps us awaken to our own natural rhythms. Like the seasons, our natural rhythms also have unique qualities, attributes, essences, and tendencies that, when understood and synchronized, help us to maintain a healthy mind, body, and spirit.

Identifying and understanding the patterns of your internal seasons will help you deepen your Slow Beauty practice, be more accepting of yourself, and will connect you with your inner rhythm. For each season, we will concentrate on two main qualities:

Goal: helps us identify what exactly we're aiming for during this season

Obstacles: roadblocks associated with each season

Imagine yourself a dancer, fluid and graceful, as you make, taste, feel, move, and touch your way through the seasons according to your personal natural rhythm, designing your inner life, and your personal standard of beauty.

AYURVEDIC CONSTITUTIONS

In the Ayurvedic tradition, constitutions (also known as *doshas*) are the total composition of an individual's mind, body, and emotional makeup. There are three different types of doshas, each of which is associated with an element: *vatta* (air, space), *pitta* (fire), and *kapha* (earth and water). An Ayurvedic practitioner will use various techniques to assess you, such as listening to your pulse, checking your tongue and eyes, and considering your body type. When you are out of balance, Ayurvedic techniques can be recommended for your dosha to help you return to a state of equilibrium.

Winter

Come sit by the hearth, tend the fire, and feel its warmth. Associated with shorter days, less light, more quiet, and breezes that are cooler and drier, winter brings with it a sharpness and a crispness. Winter embodies a distinct level of silence. The birds don't chirp, and many animals change color, migrate, and hibernate. For us humans, too, winter is a time for hibernation, withdrawing (although not *too* much), and, with this, a time for reflection and envisioning.

It may be cold on the outside during the winter months, but it is warm and cozy inside, where we retreat and withdraw. We can accomplish this by keeping our inner furnace stoked with the assistance of warming foods, movements, thoughts, and feelings. Winter is a time for being intentional and purposeful, and offers us the opportunity to gain more clarity and transparency. In the winter, we can cultivate depth and willpower. We are producing heat, through our diet, movements, breathing, thoughts, and beauty rituals.

In the Chinese tradition, winter is associated with the element of water; in the Ayurvedic tradition it is associated with the constitutions of *kapha* and *vatta*.

Goal: WARMING

Obstacles: melancholy, heavy, uninspired

Spring

This season is about complete rebirth and a flurry of activity. In the springtime, everything is growing and flowing. It is the season of renewal, of new beginnings, of birth. Renewal buzzes in the air as everything awakens from the slumber of the winter season. Bees are busy pollinating, flowers are blooming, new life is springing up everywhere. In this season we feel inspired and have the opportunity to re-engage in our creative life. Spring is full of joy as excitement blossoms around us. The pastel palette of spring reflects the nurturing softness of the season; it is a caring, supportive, and gently loving season. A season of lightheartedness. We awaken in the spring through our diet, our movements, our breath, our thoughts, and our beauty rituals.

In the Chinese tradition, spring is associated with the element of wood; in Ayurveda it is associated with the constitution of *kapha*.

Goal: EXPANSIVENESS

Obstacles: sluggishness, laziness, lackluster, rigidity, negativity, brain fog

Summer

Step into a self-confident, but dreamy state. As the sunniest time of the year, summer is all about the intensity of light. Associated with fun and freedom, the days are brighter and longer, the colors are more intense, we dress a bit lighter. Nature feels very much alive—birds chirp, pollen is spread around, and fireflies flutter as the sun sets. There is a feeling of celebration, reward, happiness, and fulfillment. The psychology of summer is passion, courage, excitement, and self-confidence. Caring for ourself is passionate and courageous. Stand in the self-confidence of summer. Feel the excitement deeply.

Summer is represented by the element of fire in the world of Chinese medicine, and *pitta* in Ayurveda.

Goal: MODERATION

Obstacles: frustration, inflammation, intolerance, perfectionism, being critical or judgmental

Fall

Release for the sake of inner strength. The sight of trees beginning to change colors in the fall is breathtaking. When the leaves finally fall from the trees, it is pure poetry. There is a distinct scent in the air that is crisp and slightly wet, and the air feels cleaner. Mimicking the falling leaves, this time of year is about letting go of that which no longer serves you, releasing what is now unnecessary. Fall is characteristic of self-discipline, structure, organization, and a deep inner strength, as we rake leaves and prepare for the long winter ahead of us, finding solace in the knowledge that spring will come again, and all will be renewed. Fall also speaks of refinement as the cooling temperatures offer us the opportunity to go within both literally and figuratively, to clean out the emotional toxins that have piled up from the previous season. The wind often picks up in the fall, so we want to watch out for imbalances associated with higher levels of worry and concern. The emotions of sadness and grief may also be "kicked up" by the winds.

Fall is associated with the element of air in Chinese medicines, and *vatta* in Ayurveda.

Goal: LETTING GO

Obstacles: Holding on to that which no longer serves us, anxiety, worry, stress, tension

taste: intentional, intuitive eating

We can raise our consciousness through the foods we consume. Here you will find recommendations and suggestions to begin your journey toward eating more consciously.

As part of the Slow Beauty practice, we increase the foods in our diet that make us feel more lively and alive and remove those that no longer serve us. This may sound daunting, but it's not. You will find that as your consciousness raises and you feel better, you will continue to shed layer after layer.

The idea is to choose foods that make us feel energetic and that have a calming or uplifting influence. When we eat foods that make us feel heavy and lethargic, then we feel heavy and lethargic. This feeling has a tendency to leak into our thoughts as well. Food affects our mood and our behaviors. Oftentimes, the "comfort" foods we seek out in moments of stress and anxiety do us more harm than good. Sure, there might be a momentary sensation of comfort but, in the long run, there are the side effects. These "comfort" foods are actually "numbing" foods. They may temporarily relieve whatever emotional symptoms we are experiencing, but they are ultimately distracting us from getting to the root of our problems

and ridding ourself of them once and for all.

Instead of using food to numb ourself and combat our emotions, let's start using it as a gentle way to nourish our body so that it doesn't have to work overtime. In doing this, we will give our body a break from the taxing digestive process that comes with foods that don't agree with us, that are inflammatory, that have no nutritious benefit, or that are not actually food.

Utilize the recipes in this chapter when you feel your body needs a little break. Each of these recipes is light and nourishing in its own way, both for your body and for your soul. They are simple, delicious, uncomplicated, classic, and whole. They are Slow Beauty in action, working for us on the deepest level, from the inside out, purifying, removing toxins, and elevating our consciousness.

Together, we'll get back to basics with simple foods and recipes that offer nutritional and medicinal benefits *and* are pleasurable to taste. That's right: these two things don't have to be mutually exclusive. Life contains so many health risks, and eating well helps us to minimize these risks. When we have an understanding of the key benefits of pomelo, turmeric, or carrot, we can begin to shift

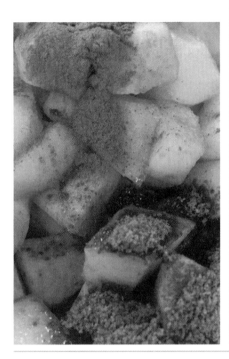

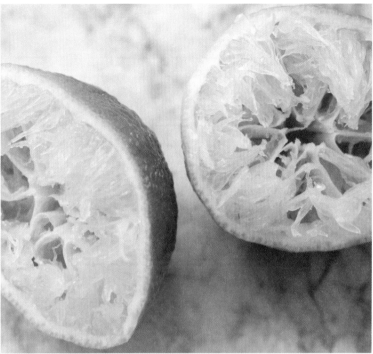

our mind-set from one of simply sustaining ourself to one of truly nourishing ourself. There is a bit of a learning curve in the beginning of this process, but once we understand how various foods benefit us, we can move from mindful eating to intuitive eating. The objective is to get to the point where our body speaks to us and we intuitively know that we need more potassium. Each of the ingredients in these recipes has a specific purpose and intention.

The number of benefits packed into natural foods is mind-bending. As we move through these recipes, I will list as many of the benefits as possible, but will nonetheless surely miss some, if not many. The idea here is to zero in on and familiarize yourself with some of a given ingredient's key benefits.

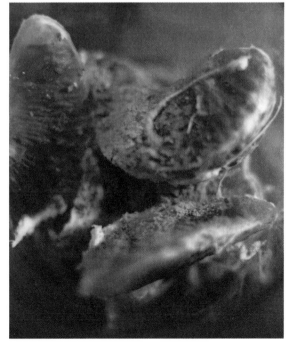

I have tried to find a balance between using accessible ingredients and introducing some that you may not be as familiar with so you can reap their benefits as well! The point here, though, is not to send you on a wild goose chase. None of the ingredients listed in this section should be so obscure that they're not available at Whole Foods or a similar market in your area, or online retailers.

With all of that in mind, I'm so excited to share some of my favorite nourishing recipes that are timeless, rather than trendy. They are meant to nourish from the inside and make us look good on the outside. Each of them contains a combination of ingredients meant to appropriately moderate energy levels for the particular season or phase you are in at any given point in time and to have a balancing effect on the central nervous system.

seasonal teas

The practice of making tea is wonderfully ceremonial. We slow down to wait as the water comes to a boil. The ingredients we work with are aromatic and beautiful to behold. There is more waiting as the ingredients steep, and the tea comes to the proper temperature for us to drink it.

Of course, there are very formal ways to experience tea. In the Slow Beauty practice, our personal "tea ceremonies" are definitely elevated, but not formalized. This practice is elevated because we can approach both making and drinking tea as a ritual. We can be intentional and mindful of the multisensory experience that includes scent, touch, taste, and sight.

You can bring as much or as little to this ceremony as you wish. It can be as minimal or as elaborate as you would like it to be. You really don't need any special equipment, or teacups—simply use what you have in your home. If you choose to have special tea accessories, that is also fine. There are beautiful collectibles out there that, for some of us, may add to our experience. But that is entirely up to you.

What I *do* recommend is that you use a combination of fresh and dried herbs and flowers to create these teas so you can enjoy the tactile, aesthetic part of the experience.

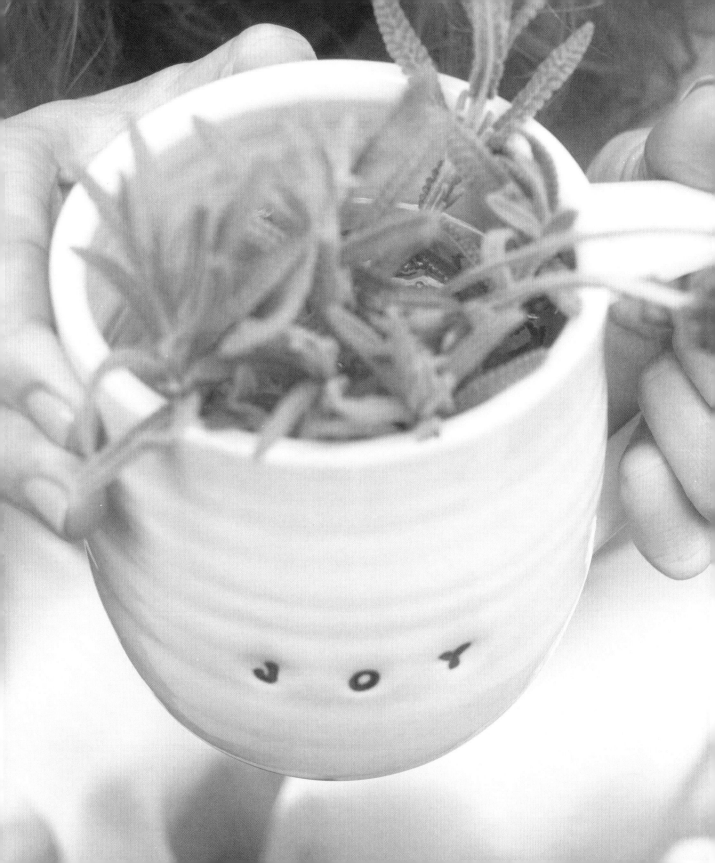

proper digestion winter tea

THIS TEA IS SIMULTANEOUSLY CALMING AND INVIGORATING, WHICH MAY seem somewhat contradictory. This winter tea will stoke your inner fire while also calming your central nervous system.

Chamomile is a healing, daisylike flower known for reducing inflammation, alleviating cold symptoms, and reducing stress. Ginger contains gingerol, which is also anti-inflammatory, aids circulation and digestion, and warms us up from the inside. And, finally, peppercorn not only adds an extra kick, but is also good for the brain and gut, regulates the mood, and is detoxifying.

MAKES FOUR 8-OUNCE CUPS

1 tablespoon dried chamomile flowers (no stems) or loose-leaf dried chamomile

1 teaspoon grated fresh ginger

4 peppercorns

32 ounces boiling water

I recommend using a teapot with an infuser for this recipe. Place the chamomile, ginger, and peppercorns in the infuser. Pour the boiling water into the teapot. Cover and let the tea steep for 5 to 7 minutes. Pour and serve.

pure poetry spring tea

THIS WILD, BOUNTIFUL TEA REFLECTS THE JOY OF SPRING. IT'S MOOD-BOOSTING, *memory-enhancing, and nurturing.*

Lavender not only smells delicious, but it also improves our mood, reduces stress and inflammation, and promotes a good night's sleep (although it may be consumed at any time of day). Basil is an adaptogen, which is a substance with ingredients that help us "smooth out" or normalize our bodily functions due to its ability to help the body adapt the stress being experienced into something more balanced. Basil combats stress, fights depression, improves memory, and serves as a tonic for our nerves. Olive oil is downright magical! It's loaded with antioxidants that help protect our heart, it enhances weight loss, and can even reduce pain.

If you'd like to take a more DIY approach to this tea, both lavender and basil are fairly easy to grow in your garden. Otherwise, fresh lavender and basil should be readily available at your local farmers' market. Simply wash the herbs in a colander, then pat them dry.

MAKES FOUR 8-OUNCE CUPS

1 tablespoon fresh lavender

1 tablespoon fresh basil

32 ounces boiling water

1 drop extra-virgin olive oil

I recommend using a teapot with an infuser for this recipe. Place the lavender and basil in the infuser. Pour the boiling water into the teapot. Cover and let the tea steep for 5 to 7 minutes. Pour. Garnish with a drop of olive oil to serve.

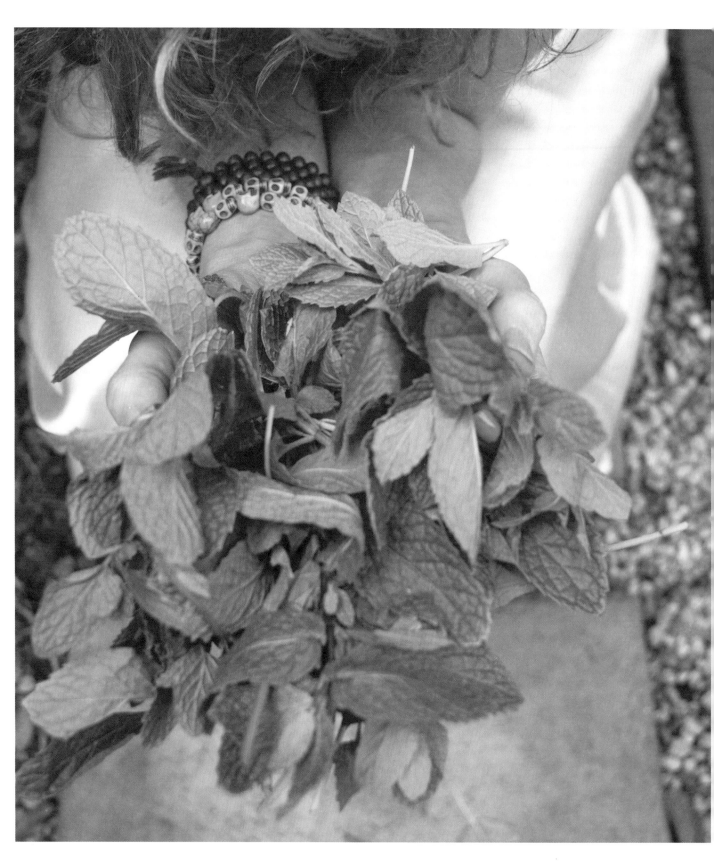

vibrant mint summer tea

THIS SIMPLE TEA WILL LEAVE YOU FEELING COOL, CALM, AND REFRESHED. MINT IS *packed with phytonutrients, which help improve overall wellness, not to mention antioxidants. It boosts immunity, freshens breath, relaxes both the body and mind, and facilitates digestion.*

MAKES FOUR 8-OUNCE CUPS

1 handful fresh mint

1 teaspoon grated orange rind

32 ounces boiling water

1 teaspoon date sugar (optional)

I recommend using a teapot with an infuser for this recipe. Place the mint and orange rind in the infuser. Pour the boiling water into the teapot. Cover and let the tea steep for 5 to 7 minutes. Pour and serve, stirring in date sugar to sweeten, if desired.

classic turmeric fall tea

THIS SILKY TEA STIMULATES, NOURISHES, SOOTHES, AND ENERGIZES. IT'S STACKED *with nutrients. Turmeric, a medicinal herb, is a powerful anti-inflammatory and strong antioxidant. Black pepper nicely complements it because it helps our body absorb the curcumin that is found in turmeric, which is a potent anti-inflammatory. Coconut milk provides us with immediate energy, prevents heart disease and cancer, improves brain function, burns fat, and builds muscle. As if that's not enough, coconut milk takes it a step further, providing us with electrolytes and combatting fatigue.*

MAKES TWO 4-OUNCE CUPS

1 tablespoon ground turmeric

1 teaspoon date sugar

1 tablespoon plus ¼ teaspoon hot water

½ cup coconut milk

1 cup water

1 (½-inch) piece fresh ginger, thinly sliced

2 pinches of freshly ground black pepper

½ teaspoon raw honey (optional)

In a small bowl, combine the turmeric, date sugar, and hot water, then whisk them into a paste. In a saucepan, whisk together the coconut milk, the cup of water, the ginger, 1 pinch of the pepper, and the turmeric paste. Bring the mixture to a light boil, then lower the heat to low and allow it to simmer for 7 minutes. Remove the saucepan from the heat, cover it, and allow it to sit for 10 minutes. Strain and serve warm. Add the remaining pinch of pepper to garnish. Add honey to sweeten, if desired.

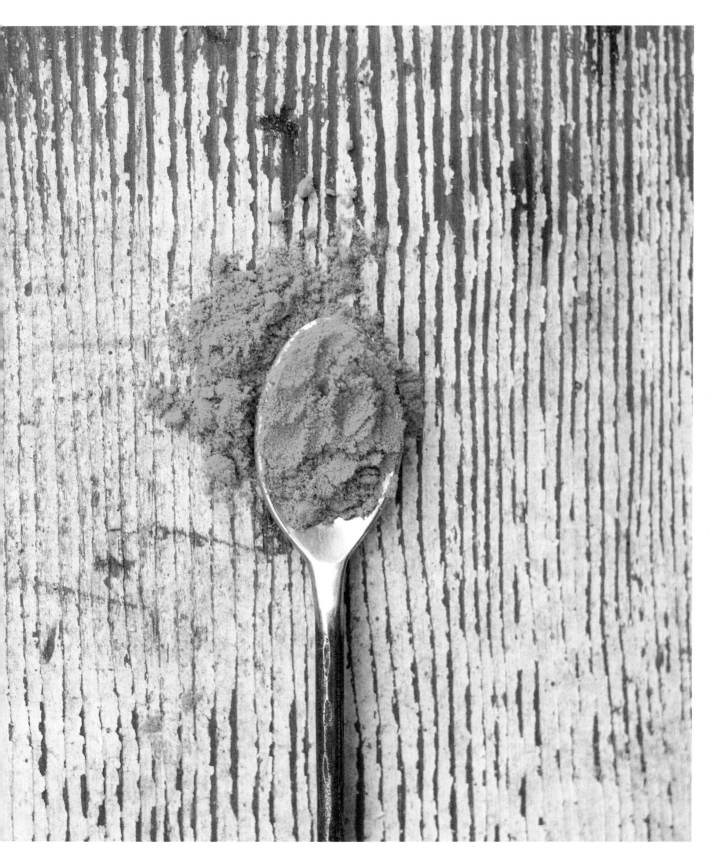

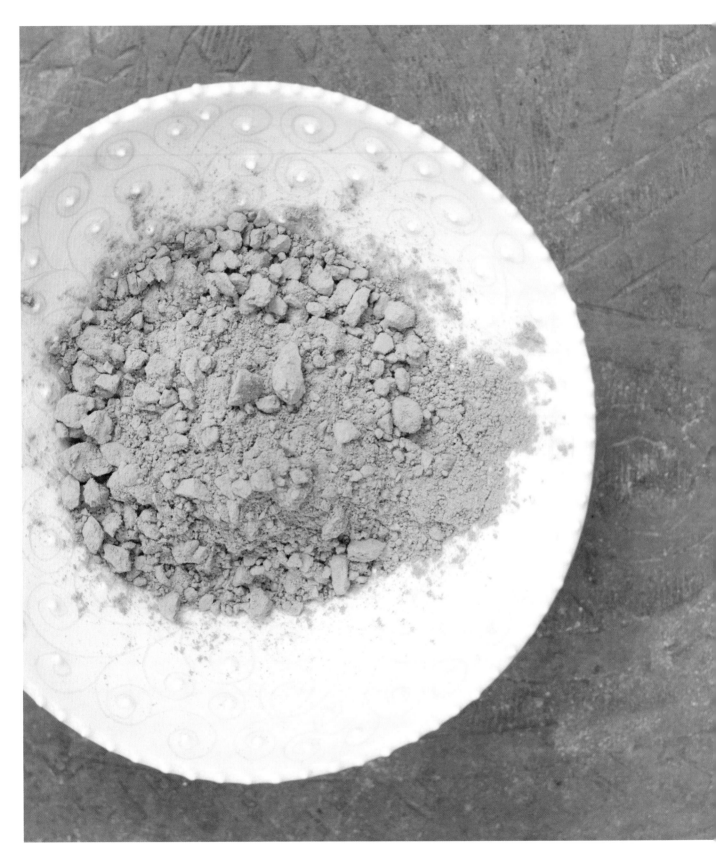

all-season classic matcha tea latte

THIS POTENT TEA CALMS, DETOXIFIES, ENHANCES MEMORY, AND BOOSTS ENERGY. *In addition to all the benefits that almond milk provides—such as glowing skin, strong bones, and heart health—matcha adds its superstar properties to the mix. Matcha is a potent antioxidant; enhances our sense of calm; boosts memory and concentration; increases metabolism, energy, and endurance; and increases blood flow and oxygen to the skin.*

MAKES ONE 6-OUNCE CUP

2 teaspoons matcha tea powder

2 tablespoons hot water

6 ounces almond milk

Heat a small bowl by pouring boiled water into it, then discard the water.

Sift the matcha tea into the heated bowl, then whisk it with the hot water to create a paste. In a saucepan over low heat, warm the almond milk. Add the matcha tea paste and, then whisk all the ingredients together. Simmer on low heat for 2 to 3 minutes. Remove the saucepan from the heat, then pour and serve.

seasonal soups

Soups are an experience in flavor, texture, and aroma. They are also a great way to obtain healthy satisfaction. The soups included here are all rich in vitamins and minerals, high in nutrient density, and low in energy density (meaning we get lots of key nutrients through a low amount of calories). Get ready to dive in and enjoy!

back to my roots winter soup

THIS WINTER SOUP WILL WARM AND SOOTHE YOU WITH A BOWLFUL OF BENEFITS. *It includes a rich mix of herbs that do everything from relieving muscle pain, improving memory, and boosting immunity to promoting hair growth, improving mood, and slowing aging. The root veggies in this soup will help you keep growing young, too, by providing a boost of vitamins that improve skin elasticity, prevent wrinkles and fine lines, and increase bone health.*

MAKES EIGHT 8-OUNCE BOWLS

3 tablespoons extra-virgin olive oil

1 cup diced yellow onion

3 garlic cloves, finely chopped

1¾ cups peeled and diced golden beet

1 medium-size red potato, diced, skin on

1 celery root, peeled and diced

1 cup diced carrot

4 cups water

2 vegetable bouillon cubes, crushed

½ teaspoon salt

¼ teaspoon freshly ground black pepper

Heat the olive oil in a soup pot over medium heat, then sauté the onion and garlic for 5 to 7 minutes, or until they're clear. Add the beet, potato, celery root, and carrot and heat for 3 to 4 minutes. Add the water and bring it to a boil. Once the water is boiling, add the crushed vegetable bouillon cubes and then lower the heat to a simmer. Add the salt and pepper. Cover the pot and allow the soup to simmer for 30 minutes, or until all the vegetables are soft. Transfer the soup to a blender and blend on medium speed until smooth. Serve.

go green spring soup

JUST AS SPRING RENEWS US, SO DOES THIS SOUP! PARSLEY IS KNOWN AS A *"chemoprotective" food, which helps neutralize such carcinogens as benzopyrenes, is rich in antioxidants, and keeps the heart healthy. Spinach supports our bones, improves eye health, and also boosts our energy for that one-two punch. As for chard, it's one of those do-it-all foods. It regulates blood sugar, prevents various types of cancer, improves digestion, detoxifies the body, and strengthens brain function. Moringa powder is an antioxidant, rich in amino acids, and supports brain health, too. I like to drink this soup first thing in the morning as part of my breakfast. Feel free to go back for seconds. Your body and brain will thank you!*

MAKES FOUR 6-OUNCE CUPS

1 tablespoon extra-virgin olive oil

½ cup chopped onion

¼ teaspoon minced jalapeño pepper

¼ teaspoon moringa powder

1 cup chopped fresh spinach

1 tablespoon finely chopped fresh basil

1 tablespoon finely chopped fresh cilantro

1 cup chopped fresh parsley

4 large chard stalks, stemmed and chopped

1 cup low-sodium vegetable broth

1 cup water

1 low-sodium vegetable bouillon cube

¼ teaspoon salt

2 pinches of freshly ground black pepper

In a 3-quart pot, heat the olive oil on medium heat and then add the onion, garlic, and jalapeño and sauté for 2 to 3 minutes, then add the moringa powder. Sauté all together until the onions are clear. Add the spinach, basil, cilantro, parsley, and chard and let steam for approximately 1 minute, then add the vegetable broth and water. Mix together and bring to a boil. When boiling, add the vegetable bouillon cube, salt, and black pepper. Lower the heat and simmer, stirring occasionally, for about 10 minutes or until all the vegetables are soft. Serve. Enjoy.

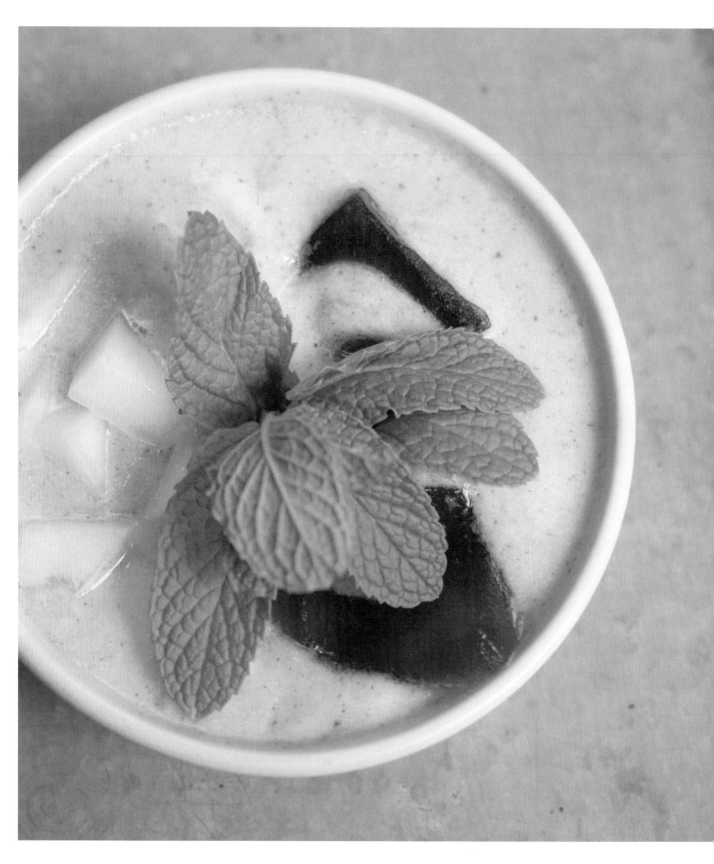

the birth of cool melon summer soup

WHEN WE THINK OF SOUP, WE OFTEN THINK OF A PIPING-HOT BOWL TO WARM *us up on a cold winter's day. But soup is also great for cooling. And this oh-so-simple melon soup will do precisely that, and so much more. Keep your energy up with Medjool dates, and rejuvenate your skin and keep it shining and healthy with lime juice. Your mood will remain in check, thanks to hibiscus, which also calms the nervous system, protects the liver, and guards against inflammation.*

MAKES FOUR 12-OUNCE BOWLS

2 hibiscus tea bags

16 ounces boiling water

1 large honeydew melon: carve out ¾ of the flesh to use in the soup, cube ¼ of the remaining flesh and set aside, for garnish

3 Medjool dates, pitted

2 teaspoons minced fresh ginger

¼ cup freshly squeezed lime juice

12 large fresh mint leaves

2 pinches Celtic sea salt

Place the tea bags in a 32-ounce glass measuring cup. Pour the boiling water over the tea bags. Steep in the hot water for 4 to 5 minutes, until the water turns red. Reserve 8 ounces of the hibiscus tea, allowing it to cool to room temperature, then place it in the refrigerator to chill. Pour the remaining hibiscus tea evenly into an ice cube tray and freeze.

Combine the honeydew, dates, ginger, lime juice, 11 of the mint leaves, and the salt, 2 hibiscus tea ice cubes, and chilled hibiscus tea in a high-speed blender. Blend on medium to high speed for 20 to 30 seconds, or until the soup is smooth.

Pour the soup into bowls to serve immediately. Garnish with cubed honeydew melon, the remaining mint leaf, and a hibiscus ice cube. Drink up and cool down!

optimistic squash fall soup

THIS SOUP IS NOT ONLY A BEAUTY TO BEHOLD DUE TO ITS GORGEOUS AUTUMNAL *orange hue, but it is also packed with beautiful and highly beneficial ingredients. Squash is great for the heart, high in fiber, and good for the bones, plus the flesh and seeds of the squash contain zinc, which is linked to increasing bone density. The grapeseed oil used as one of the garnishes contains antioxidants and anti-inflammatories.*

MAKES EIGHT 8-OUNCE BOWLS

1 medium-size butternut squash, peeled and cubed

1 tablespoon coconut oil

2 shallots, thinly diced

2 garlic cloves, minced

Pinch of Celtic sea salt

Pinch of freshly ground black pepper

¼ teaspoon ground dried rosemary

1 (14-ounce) can light coconut milk

2 cups vegetable broth

2 tablespoons coconut sugar

Raw, sprouted pumpkin seeds, for garnish

Grapeseed oil, for garnish

Chopped shallot, for garnish

Coconut flakes, for garnish

Remove the seeds from the butternut squash, then wash the seeds, remove any remaining squash flesh, and set the seeds aside.

Heat a soup pot over medium heat. Add the coconut oil, shallots, and garlic, allowing them to sauté for 2 to 4 minutes, stirring often. Add the squash, salt, pepper, and rosemary. Then, add the coconut milk, vegetable broth, and coconut sugar. Bring the soup to a boil over medium heat, then lower the heat to low, cover the pot, and allow the soup to simmer for approximately 15 minutes, or until the squash is tender.

Transfer the soup to a blender and puree on high speed until it is creamy and smooth. Return it to the pot to warm on low heat for 5 to 7 minutes.

Heat a small sauté pan on medium heat. Lower the heat to low, then place the butternut squash seeds in the pan to toast for 3 to 5 minutes, or until golden.

To serve, garnish the soup with toasted squash seeds, pumpkin seeds, a drizzle of grapeseed oil, a sprinkle of chopped shallot, and coconut flakes.

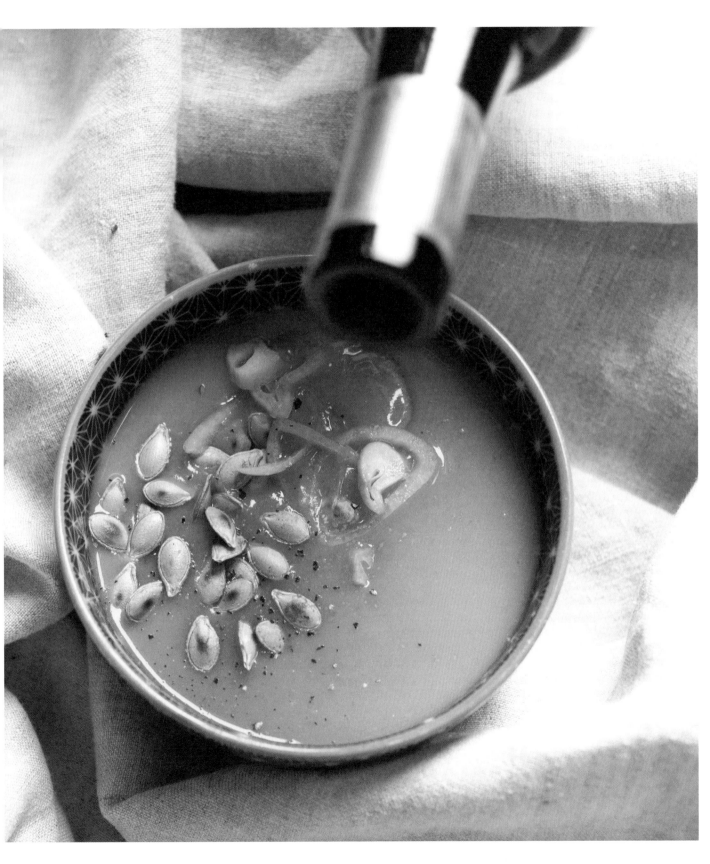

stress-busting all-season vegetable broth

THE KEY INGREDIENT OF THIS VEGETABLE BROTH IS POTASSIUM, WHICH IS DERIVED *from a combination of many of the vegetables in the recipe. Potassium is greatly helpful for those suffering from undesirable mental states, such as anxiety and stress. It is considered a powerful stress-buster and, therefore, ensures the efficient mental performance of the human body. Not only this, but potassium can also help regulate various hormones in our body, such as cortisol and adrenaline, excess amounts of which can be quite detrimental to a wide array of our body's systems. When it is combined with the variety of folates, fiber, flavonoids, vitamins, and minerals also included in this soup, you'll feel more energized and balanced.*

MAKES 64 OUNCES

1 large onion

1 large parsnip

3 large carrots

4 celery ribs

1 leek, white and pale green part, and 3 green stalks

3 large white mushrooms (with stems)

2 garlic cloves, smashed

4 to 5 thyme sprigs

Leaves from 1 bunch parsley

1 bay leaf

1 teaspoon whole peppercorns

1 teaspoon ground turmeric

1 teaspoon smoked paprika

1 teaspoon sea salt

Roughly chop all the vegetables. Place them in a stockpot. Fill the pot with just enough water to cover the vegetables. Add the garlic, thyme, parsley, bay leaf, peppercorns, turmeric, paprika, and salt. Cover and heat over medium-high heat to just under a boil. Lower the heat and, stirring occasionally, simmer for 1 hour.

Allow the soup to cool, then remove the vegetables with a slotted spoon. Pour the rest of the stock through a strainer. Discard the solids. Use the broth immediately or cool and freeze it in airtight plastic containers or freezer bags. It will keep in the refrigerator for 3 to 4 days. I like to drink this like a tea and I also freeze this broth to use as vegetable stock in other soup recipes.

seasonal juices

Fresh juices are packed with vitamins, minerals, phytonutrients, and enzymes. They're easy to digest, increase energy, and give you access to a wider variety of fruit and vegetables you may not usually consume. Oh, and there is one compote here, to mix things up a bit.

slow-aging bitters winter juice

THIS POWERFUL JUICE HAS A TON OF INGREDIENTS THAT WARD OFF DISEASE TO HELP *us live a long, vibrant, healthy life. Thanks to its high amounts of vitamin C and antioxidants, even a small glass of freshly squeezed grapefruit can help detoxify the liver by flushing out carcinogens and other toxins. Also high in vitamin C as well as containing spermadine, pomelos, found at Whole Foods Market during the winter months, help restore skin cells, increase longevity, and slow the aging process. As for parsley, well, it's more than just a garnish. In fact, it's a superfood. Parsley keeps the heart healthy, can help prevent oxygen-based damage to cells, and rids the body of free radicals that play a role in the development and progression of diseases, including everything from cancer to diabetes to asthma.*

MAKES ONE 8-OUNCE GLASS

½ pomelo

1 small to medium-size grapefruit

1 handful fresh parsley

Pinch of freshly ground black pepper, for garnish

Dash of agave syrup, for garnish (optional)

Place the pomelo, grapefruit, and parsley in a cold-press juicer and blend. Transfer the juice to a glass and garnish with the pepper and agave, if desired.

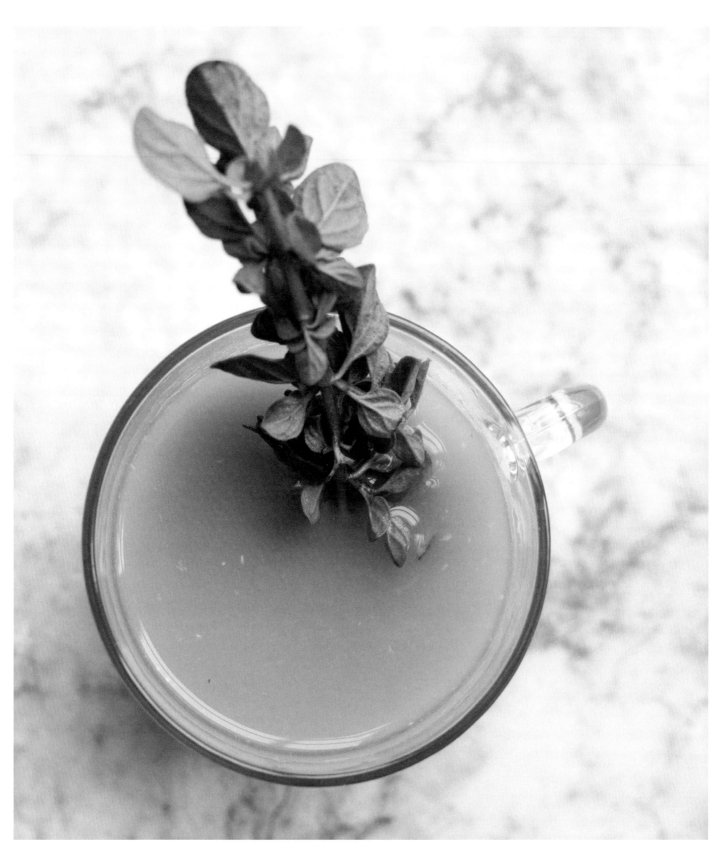

radiant immunity sour spring juice

EVEN IF THIS REFRESHING DRINK WASN'T SO INCREDIBLY GOOD FOR YOU, CHANCES *are you would still want to gulp it down. Happily, though, it's both delicious and incredibly healthy. The cucumber base—comprising 96 percent water—will keep you hydrated and fight off the heat, both inside and out. It supplies skin-friendly minerals, aids in weight loss, and cuts down cancer risk. Lemon is useful for so many things, including preventing diabetes; combatting constipation; fighting high blood pressure; and improving skin, hair, and teeth. And, finally, oregano is the granddaddy of all antioxidants—in fact, it packs a full forty-two times the punch of apples! It's also good for combatting a host of other conditions, including bloating, dandruff, acne, and toothaches, just to name a few.*

MAKES ONE 8-OUNCE GLASS

1 medium-size cucumber

1 small lemon

1 oregano sprig

1 small green tomato (if you can't find a green one, use a small red one instead)

Pinch of freshly ground black pepper, for garnish

Pinch of Celtic sea salt, for garnish

Place the cucumber, lemon, oregano, and tomato in a cold-press juicer and blend. Transfer the juice to a glass and garnish with the pepper and salt.

goodness in a glass summer juice

SUNCHOKES, ALSO KNOWN AS JERUSALEM ARTICHOKES, ARE RICH IN A FIBER *called inulin, which is a prebiotic. A prebiotic is the food the probiotic bacteria (good bacteria) in your gut needs to provide their health benefits to you. Sunchokes are also packed with iron and potassium and help the body absorb certain minerals. Basil helps reduce stress due to a phytochemical it contains, which is known to reduce cortisol, clear up the skin, and detoxify the liver. Do be aware that sunchokes may cause gas, so drink in moderation.*

MAKES ONE 4-OUNCE GLASS

4 sunchokes

2 ounces fresh basil

Place the sunchokes and basil in a cold-press juicer and blend. Transfer the juice to a glass and serve.

tastes like apple pie fall compote

OUR FALL JUICE IS ACTUALLY NOT A JUICE AT ALL, BUT A COMPOTE. *COMPOTE means "mixture" in French, and this delicious mixture originated in medieval Europe, where compotes were originally served as desserts. While compotes are certainly tasty enough to be desserts, they pack enough nutrients to be consumed at any time of day.*

MAKES TWO 8-OUNCE BOWLS

2 apples, peeled, cored, and chopped

2 pears, peeled, cored, and chopped

¼ teaspoon ground cinnamon

1½ tablespoons raw coconut sugar

4 ounces water

5 prunes

Place the apples, pears, cinnamon, coconut sugar, and water in a saucepan. Bring to a simmer and cook, stirring occasionally, for 15 to 20 minutes, until the fruit is soft. Add the prunes and simmer for 5 to 7 more minutes.

This compote may be served hot or cold. Enjoy!

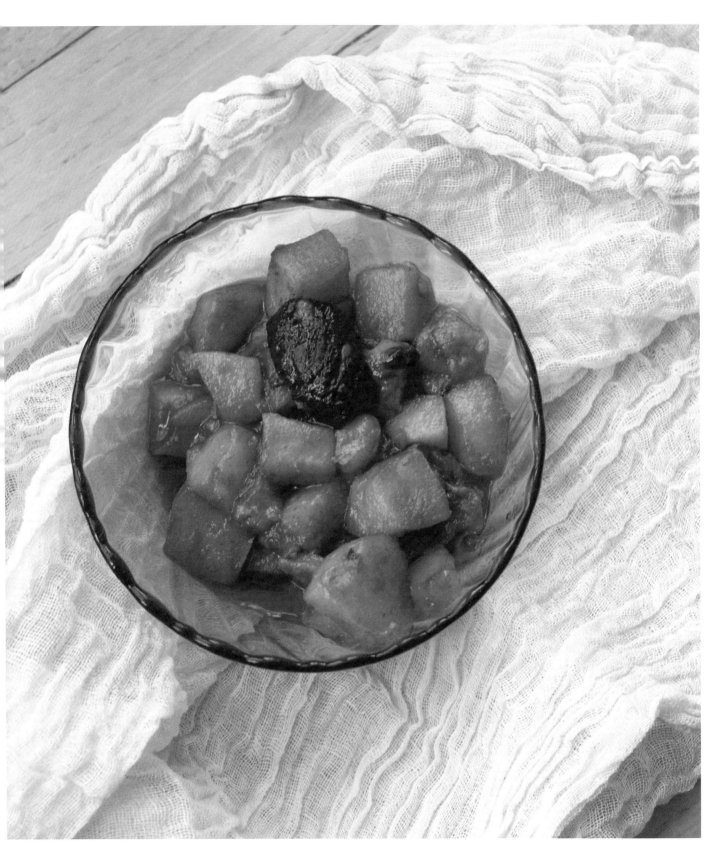

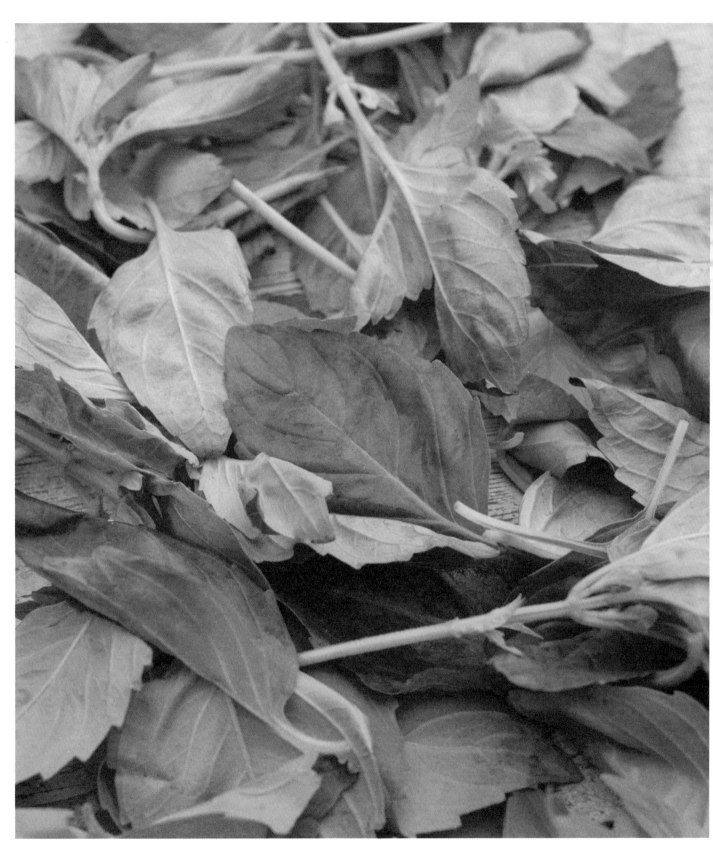

all-season glorious greens

GLORIOUS INDEED! SPINACH IS ALKALINE IN NATURE, SO IT HELPS KEEP THE PH LEVELS *of the body in balance, and is also high in protein and iron. Parsley, also high in iron, is good for the bones, and boosts the immune system with its high content of vitamin C. Beautiful basil helps to smooth out stress and anxiety, while raw garlic is excellent for brain and heart health, regulates blood pressure, and fights the common cold.*

MAKES ONE 4-OUNCE GLASS

½ cup baby spinach

¼ cup fresh parsley

7 to 8 fresh basil leaves

2 garlic cloves

Place the spinach, parsley, basil leaves, and garlic in a cold-press juicer and blend. Transfer the juice to a glass and serve.

seasonal smoothies and bowls

Smoothies and bowls are a great way to nourish your body. Not only are they nutrient-dense, but they're also detoxifying since they give your digestive system a break. Clearly, they are a great way to jump-start your day *and* they're fun to make!

almond butter pomelo winter smoothie

PERFECT FOR WINTER, THIS SMOOTHIE IS RICH IN GOOD FATS AND HIGH IN *antioxidants. Pomelo is rich in vitamin C, which will help bolster your immune system during the winter months. Turmeric, a great anti-inflammatory, works hand in hand with pepper, which helps the body absorb the effects of the turmeric.*

MAKES FOUR 6-OUNCE GLASSES

3 tablespoons almond butter

1 cup chilled chamomile tea

1 cup ice

¼ pomelo

½ teaspoon ground turmeric

1¼ cups coconut yogurt

Coconut flakes, for garnish

Pepper, for garnish

Place the almond butter, tea, ice, pomelo, turmeric, and yogurt in a blender. Blend on medium speed until all the ingredients are incorporated. Transfer the smoothie to glasses and garnish with coconut flakes and pepper, to serve.

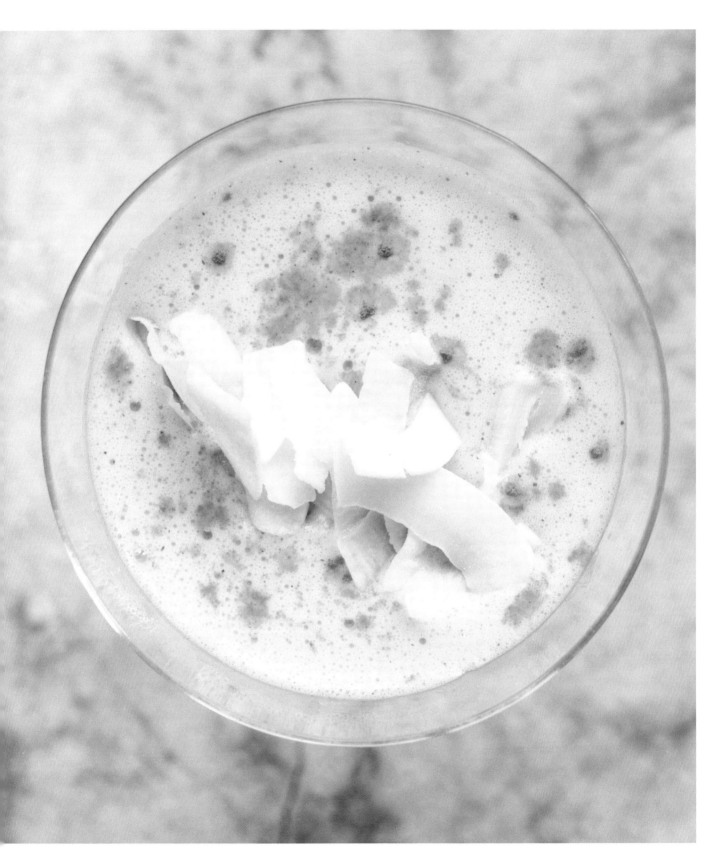

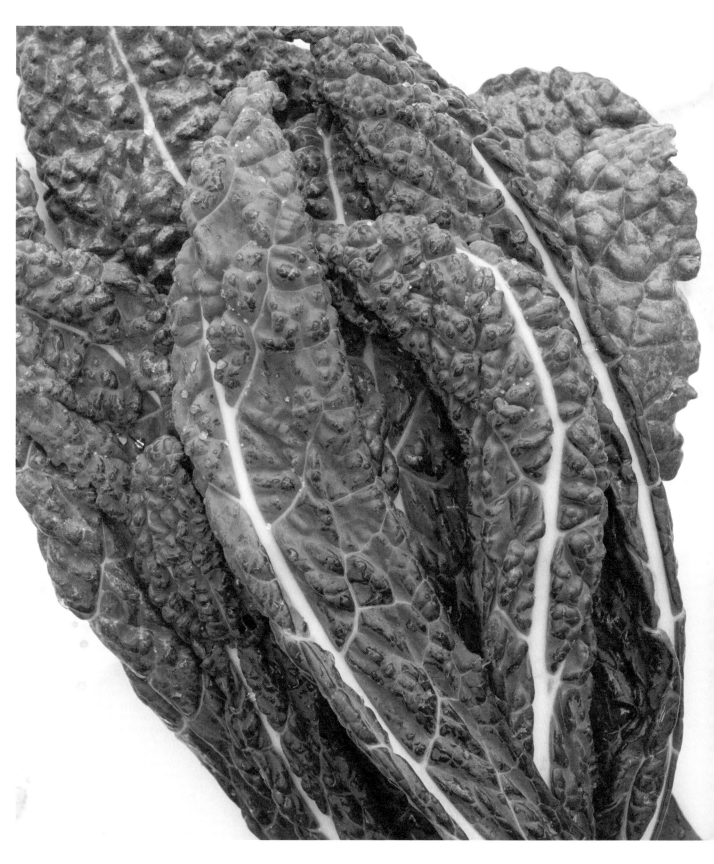

good fortune spring smoothie

PLUMS SYMBOLIZE GOOD FORTUNE IN THE CHINESE TRADITION. IN THIS RECIPE, *though, we're using the dried version of plums—prunes—instead because they contain a significantly higher amount of nutrients than do fresh plums. Apples, also a main ingredient of this smoothie, are rich in antioxidants, and are beneficial for brain and heart health. Kale is included for its high nutrient density.*

MAKES ONE 8-OUNCE GLASS

1 medium-size red apple, cored

1 tablespoon coconut yogurt

2 small pitted prunes

¼ cup prune juice

2 kale stalks, stemmed and chopped

½ cup water

½ cup ice

In a blender, combine all the ingredients. Blend on medium speed until a smooth, creamy texture is achieved. Serve and enjoy.

pure sunshine summer smoothie

IF YOU HAVEN'T TRIED SUNFLOWER SEED BUTTER YET, YOU'RE MISSING OUT. *Not only is it delicious, but it's also a great source of vitamins E, B_1, and copper. This single food protects against free radicals, helps drive the chemical reactions your cells need to function, and benefits your hair and skin! Combine this with honeydew, which packs in essential vitamins and minerals for optimal health and has lots of fiber to regulate digestion, and this smoothie will have your body humming all day long!*

MAKES ONE 16-OUNCE GLASS

1 cup seeded and cubed honeydew melon

4 tablespoons coconut yogurt

2 tablespoons sunflower butter

2 large hibiscus tea ice cubes (page 119)

1 mango, peeled, pitted, and sliced, for garnish

Place the honeydew, yogurt, sunflower butter, and ice cubes in a blender. Blend on medium speed until a smooth, creamy texture is achieved. If the smoothie is too thick, add additional ice cubes, one at a time. Garnish the smoothie with a few slices of mango, to serve.

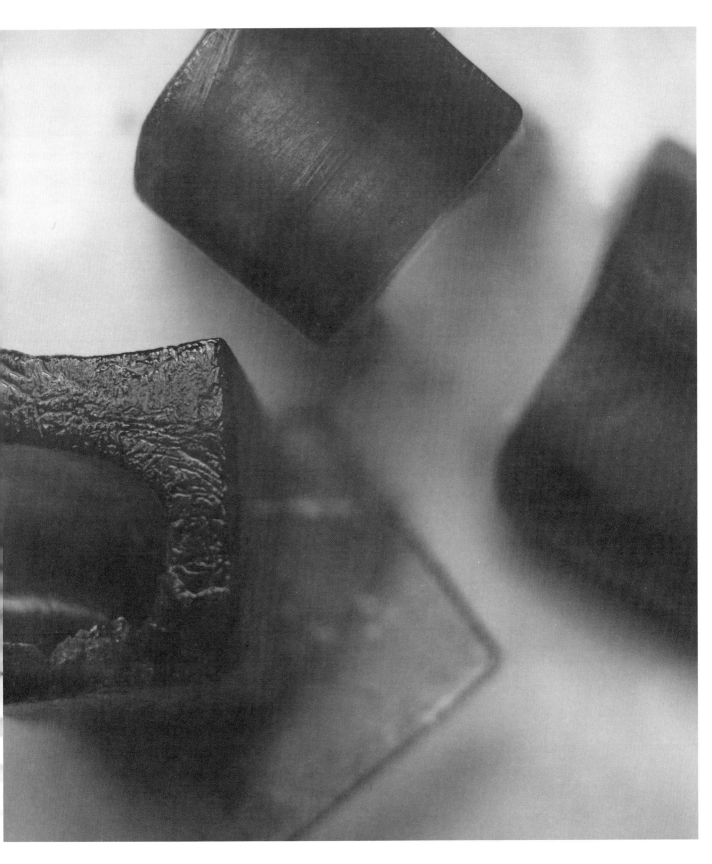

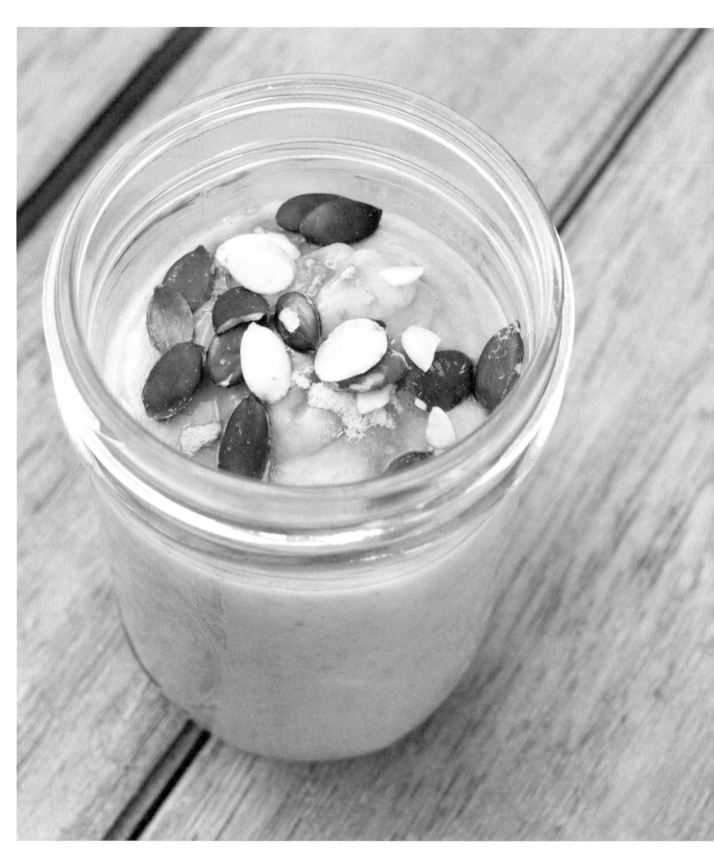

from-a-to-z fall smoothie

THIS FALL SMOOTHIE CONTAINS EVERYTHING YOU NEED, FROM A TO Z! POMEGRANATES *kick it off with antioxidants and vitamin C. Pears are a good source of dietary fiber, not to mention being jam-packed with minerals and nutrients. Figs are good for bones and heart health, as well as rich in potassium and other vitamins and minerals. Pumpkin seeds round this smoothie out as an excellent source of zinc.*

MAKES FOUR 6-OUNCE GLASSES

4 tablespoons coconut yogurt

4 pears, sliced and cored

4 figs (preferably fresh, but dried will work, if necessary)

1 tablespoon pomegranate powder

Raw pumpkin seeds, for garnish

Pomegranate powder, for garnish

Place the yogurt, pears, figs, and pomegranate powder in a blender. Blend on medium speed until all the ingredients are combined. Transfer the smoothie to glasses and garnish with pumpkin seeds and pomegranate powder.

all-season endurance smoothie

NOT ONLY DOES THIS SMOOTHIE HIT THE SPOT WITH ITS PERFECT BALANCE OF *savory and sweet, but the amount of benefits included in this single drink are almost unbelievable. It simultaneously boosts muscle strength and power; moisturizes skin from within; reduces blood pressure; increases brain power; boosts energy; balances the mood; improves sexual function; improves memory and concentration; increases metabolism; promotes a good night's sleep; bolsters immunity; and it increases feelings of bliss. I mean, talk about superpowers in a glass! Although it is not absolutely necessary, I prefer to freeze many of the ingredients in this recipe for the perfectly chilled temperature.*

MAKES ONE 12-OUNCE GLASS

8 ounces frozen organic almond milk, plus ¼ cup not frozen

1 frozen banana

3 to 4 ounces coconut water

1 teaspoon organic maca powder

1 teaspoon organic raw cacao powder

½ teaspoon ground cinnamon

Pinch of Celtic sea salt

3 to 4 Medjool dates, pitted

1 teaspoon organic green coffee powder

Cacao nibs, for garnish

Combine both the frozen and not frozen almond milk, and the banana, coconut water, maca powder, cacao powder, cinnamon, salt, dates, and green coffee powder in a blender. Mix on medium speed until a smooth consistency is achieved (you may want to pause the blender and shake the ingredients halfway through to fully incorporate).

Pour the smoothie into a glass and sprinkle cacao nibs over the top, to garnish.

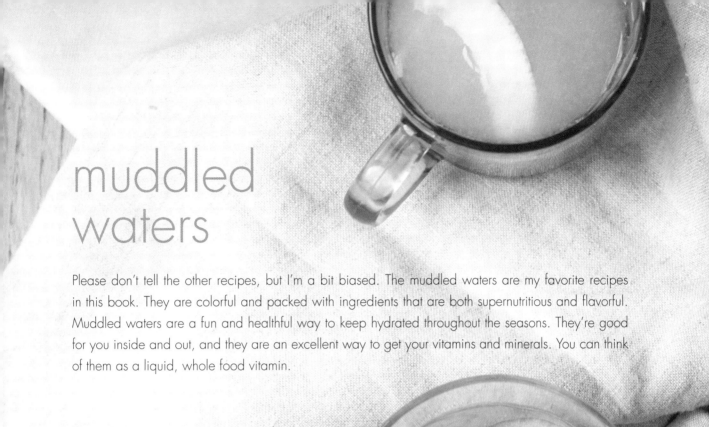

muddled
waters

Please don't tell the other recipes, but I'm a bit biased. The muddled waters are my favorite recipes in this book. They are colorful and packed with ingredients that are both supernutritious and flavorful. Muddled waters are a fun and healthful way to keep hydrated throughout the seasons. They're good for you inside and out, and they are an excellent way to get your vitamins and minerals. You can think of them as a liquid, whole food vitamin.

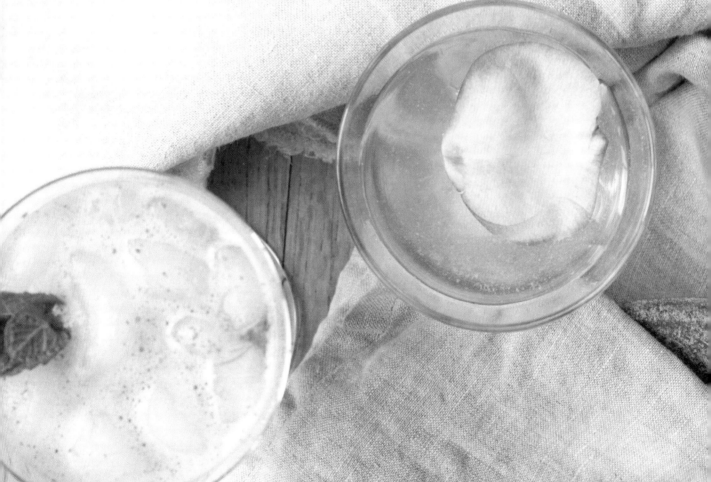

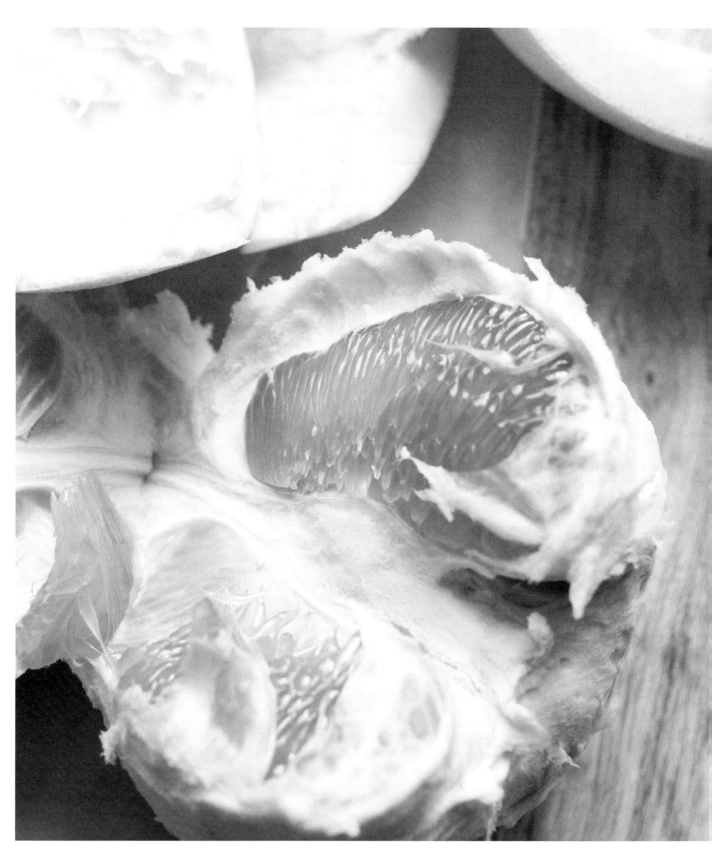

garlic-lemon drop winter water

GARLIC BOOSTS THE IMMUNE SYSTEM, HAS MEDICINAL PROPERTIES, IS HIGHLY *nutritious, contains antioxidants, and is also good for the heart. Lemon purifies, while pomelo is known to reduce the appearance of wrinkles by improving blood flow to the surface of the skin. Pomelo also increases collagen production and, in general, helps the skin look healthy.*

MAKES ONE 12-OUNCE GLASS

4 pomelo wedges

½ teaspoon garlic powder

Juice of ½ lemon

10 ounces water, at room-temperature

2 ounces boiling water

Place the pomelo wedges, garlic powder, and lemon juice in a tumbler and muddle them together. Cover the ingredients with the room-temperature water and stir. Then, add the boiling water to top off the cup and warm it up.

Allow the water to sit for a few minutes before serving so the ingredients infuse together for a more vibrant taste experience. Drink and chew all the ingredients.

rose energy spring water

ROSE ESSENTIAL OIL BOOSTS YOUR MOOD, WHILE PROBIOTICS KEEP YOUR GUT HEALTHY *and boost your immune system. Meanwhile, the alkaline water will go to work neutralizing the acidic conditions in your gut and improving your energy levels.*

MAKES ONE 4-OUNCE GLASS

4 ounces alkaline water, at room temperature

1 (.15-ounce) packet powdered probiotics

1 drop rose essential oil

Place all the ingredients in a glass and stir them all together. Drink immediately.

aloe i love you summer water

STEP IT UP THIS SUMMER WITH THIS *refreshing and rejuvenating water. Tangelos contain significant levels of folate, which makes DNA and other genetic materials. Alkaline water neutralizes acid in the bloodstream. The reparative flesh of aloe vera has internal cleansing and healing properties. Do be aware that too much aloe vera juice may cause diarrhea, so drink in moderation.*

MAKES ONE 10-OUNCE GLASS

2 to 3 tangelos or other small citrus fruit, such as mandarin oranges, peeled (and seeded, if applicable)

1 (3-inch) piece aloe vera flesh from 1 aloe vera leaf, skinned

8 ounces alkaline water

Handful of fresh mint leaves

½ teaspoon agave syrup

Ice

Combine the tangelos, aloe vera flesh, water, mint leaves, and agave in a blender and blend on high speed until the drink reaches a frothy state. Pour over ice to serve. Enjoy!

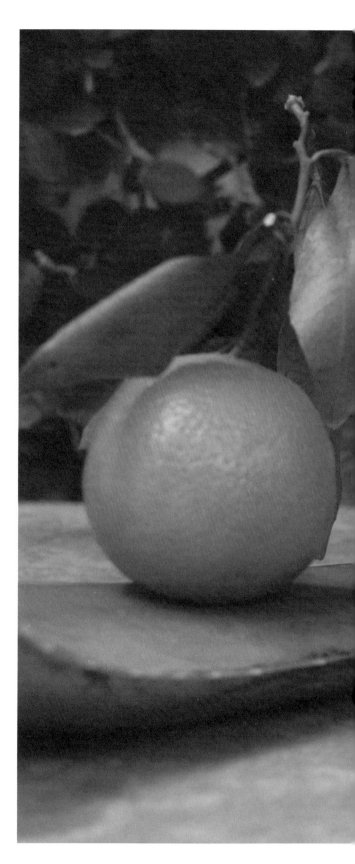

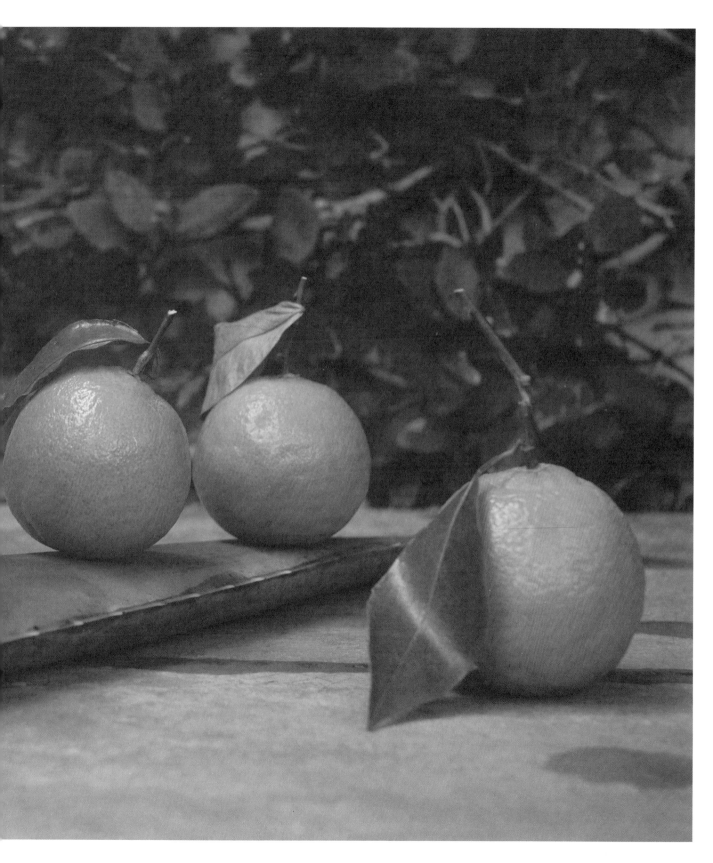

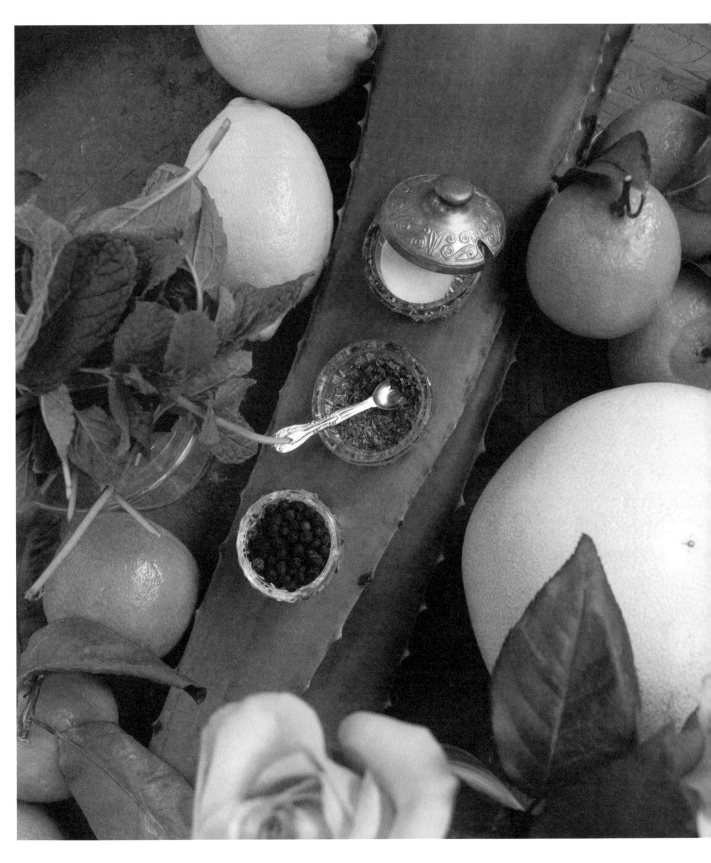

turmeric orange fall water

THIS WATER WILL MAKE YOUR ENTIRE BODY SING. BLOOD RED ORANGES CONTAIN *anthocyanin, which helps the body heal itself. Lemon purifies the skin and parsley is nutrient-dense. Turmeric is an antioxidant and pepper helps your body digest the turmeric. Drink up and feel great!*

MAKES ONE 12-OUNCE GLASS

2 to 3 wedges from a small blood red orange (any type of orange can be substituted, if preferred)

¼ teaspoon ground turmeric

Pinch of dried parsley

Juice of ½ lemon

12 ounces warm water

Freshly ground black pepper, for garnish

Parsley sprig, for garnish

Place the orange wedges, turmeric, parsley, and lemon juice in a glass. Muddle the ingredients together. Cover the mixture with the warm water. Enjoy!

hot lemon all-season water

MY GRANDMOTHER DRANK HOT WATER WITH LEMON, MY MOTHER DRANK HOT *water with lemon, and that's why I drink hot water with lemon. Many cultures around the world, including the Ayurvedic tradition, highly value this drink for its detoxifying benefits. Lemon is a panacea with so many health benefits. This superfruit is packed with numerous vitamins and minerals, it helps us shed pounds, is known to rejuvenate the skin, and helps boost the mood.*

MAKES ONE 8-OUNCE GLASS

8 ounces boiling spring water

½ lemon

Pour the boiling spring water into a glass, then squeeze the lemon into the water. Let the water stand for a few minutes to cool before serving.

feel:
remember your
beautiful body

More often than not, beauty routines focus on our face and neglect the needs of the rest of the body. This is why I'm such a big fan of spas. Spas have always focused on treating the mind, body, and spirit. They generally put a special emphasis on calming the nervous system and creating a sense of wholeness for the entire being.

The recipes in this section include the sort of scrubs, oils, soaks, and mists that spas have been using for decades to nourish the body and help us feel more connected to it. All too often, we jump out of bed and rush absent-mindedly through our morning routine, then dash out the door and into our day, completely taking our body for granted. The yummy recipes in this section are designed to create more space and time for intentional body rituals, such as daily self-massage, exfoliation, soaks, and misting. These rituals are meant to show us how to love our body just the way it is. This fourfold approach is the road to a glowing, healthy, toned, detoxed, and joyful mind, body, and soul.

In addition to making use of the recipes in this book, I also highly recommend making time to go to a spa for professional body treatments on a regular basis. It's an investment in you, your health, and your state of mind.

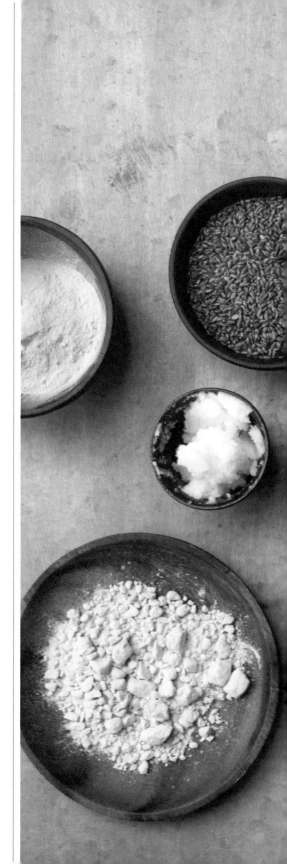

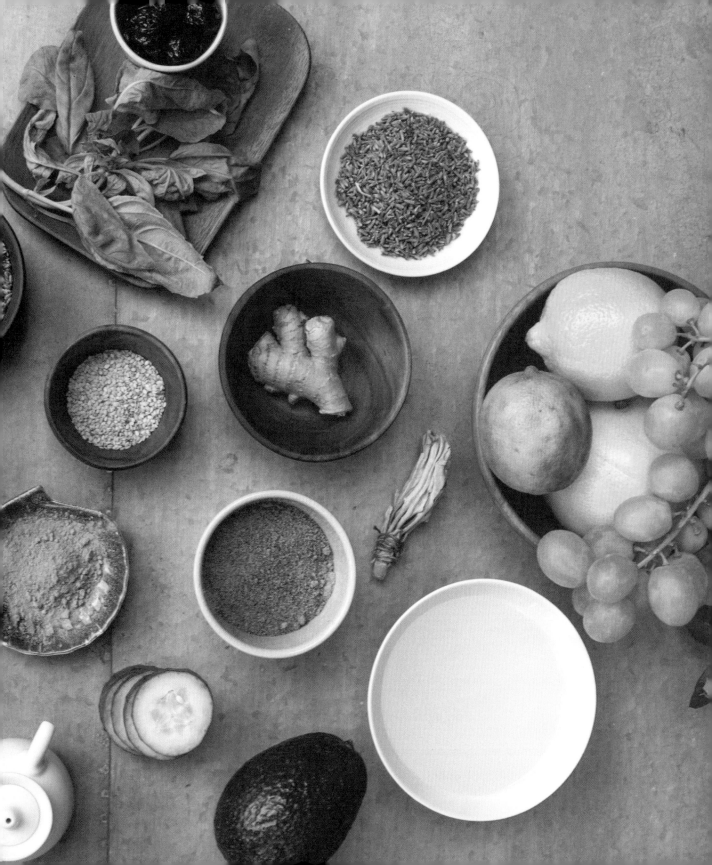

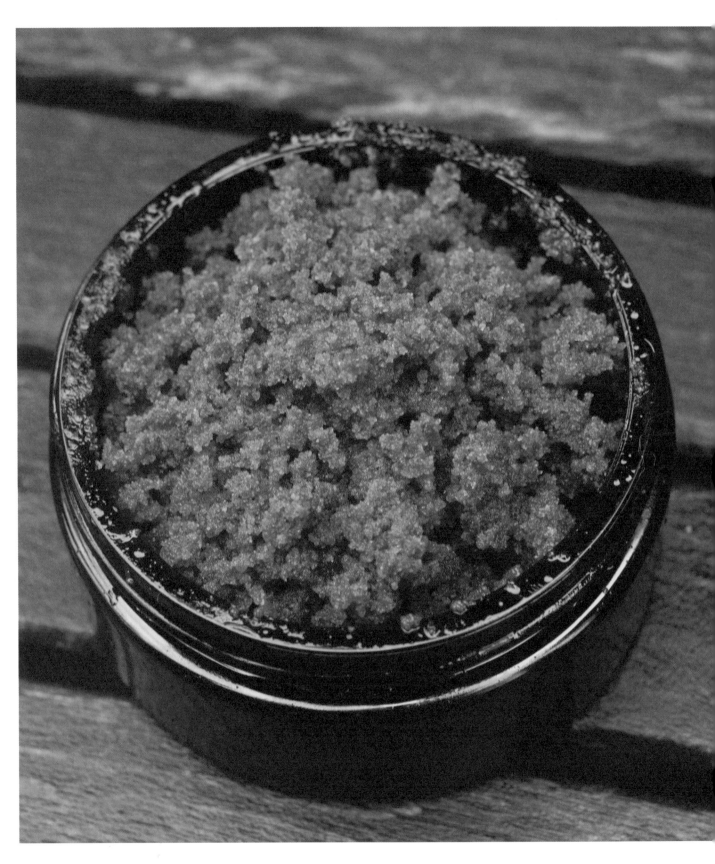

scrubs

Exfoliation is so beneficial for the skin. It sloughs off dead skin cells and increases circulation, which detoxifies the skin and leaves us with a beautiful, healthy glow. Be sure to drink lots of water on the days you exfoliate, to help generate new skin cell growth.

grapefruit, ginger, and grapeseed oil paste winter scrub

THIS SCRUB IS WET, DENSE, AND PASTY AND WHEN YOU APPLY IT TO YOUR WET SKIN, it opens up with a bright grapefruit pick-me-up and warming gingeriness. The grapeseed base allows the scrub to glide onto the skin.

I love using grapeseed oil in the winter because it is a wonderful moisturizer for combatting that dry winter skin, and also contains powerful antioxidants, which are particularly important during this time of the year. The fresh ginger warms the muscles and tones the skin, while grapefruit essential oil uplifts the mood, reduces the appearance of cellulite, and detoxifies.

Use this scrub in the shower. First wet your entire body and then begin the exfoliation process, paying special attention to dry spots, such as your elbows and feet. For winter exfoliation, use deeper pressure as you exfoliate your skin to relieve muscle tension and stimulate circulation.

MAKES 12 OUNCES

1 cup coconut sugar

2 tablespoons grated fresh ginger

4 tablespoons grapeseed oil

12 to 15 drops grapefruit essential oil

In a bowl, whisk together the sugar and ginger, then add the grapeseed oil and grapefruit essential oil. Continue to whisk until the ingredients are fully blended. Transfer to an airtight container and store at room temperature. Use within 7 days.

lavender, matcha, and avocado oil spring exfoliating powder

THIS BLEND FEELS LIKE A GENTLE BRUSH OF SOFTENING, THANKS TO THE AVOCADO OIL, *combined with a calming breath of lavender, and a wake-up call, compliments of matcha. It is best applied in small amounts, and slowly brushed onto the skin with your fingertips.*

Avocado oil has excellent moisturizing penetration qualities, and assists with repairing and softening skin. Matcha stimulates cell regeneration, contains chlorophyll, which is a powerful detoxifier, and has many antioxidants. Aromatic lavender is calming and toning.

This scrub has a drier, powderlike consistency, almost like a sand scrub. It is meant to be brushed onto dry skin in quick motions with your hand. Exfoliate toward your heart to increase the blood flow. When you've finished brushing, rinse the scrub off with warm water. Your skin will be silky smooth, and your body and mind will feel awakened and peaceful. Finish this pampering off by massaging a coat of Lemon Primrose Spring Oil (page 157) all over your body.

MAKES 8 OUNCES

1 cup coconut sugar

1½ teaspoons matcha tea powder

2 tablespoons avocado oil

5 drops lavender essential oil

In a bowl, whisk together the sugar and matcha tea until fully blended. Add the avocado oil and lavender essential oil and continue to whisk until the scrub is fully blended. Store in an airtight container at room temperature. Use within 7 days.

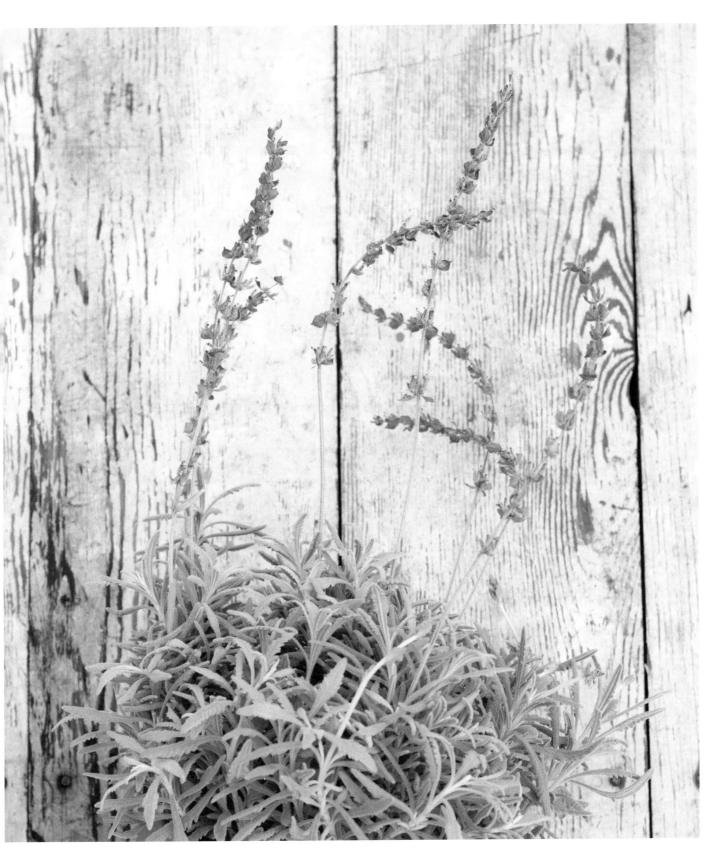

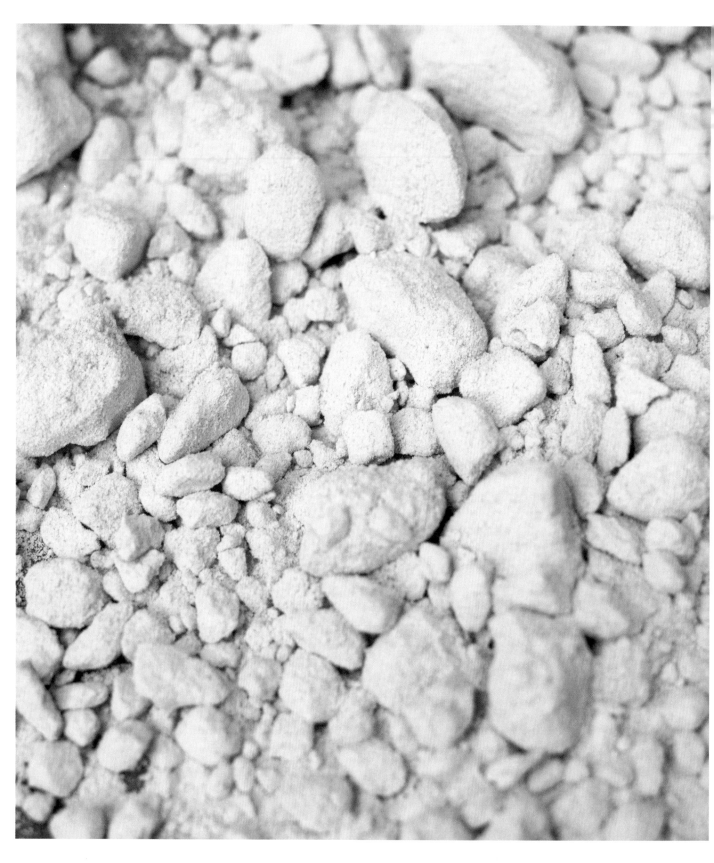

basil, maca, and sunflower summer exfoliating powder

YOU'LL LOVE THIS BRIGHT BRUSHING OF SUNFLOWERS, LUSTY MACA ROOT, AND *mineral-rich holy basil to increase endurance and smooth out stress. Like the spring scrub, this scrub has a powderlike texture and is meant to be applied in small amounts and rapidly brushed onto the skin with your fingertips to energize.*

Sunflower oil is a great ingredient to incorporate whenever you can during the summer because it prevents water loss, which makes staying hydrated that much easier! Maca powder enlivens the libido, and holy basil increases endurance and relieves joint pain. Apply this scrub in the shower prior to turning on the water. Apply it in small amounts by hand, starting from the tips of your extremities and moving upward toward your heart with quick, repetitive strokes. This is the best technique to increase detoxifying blood circulation. When you are done, rinse with warm water, towel dry, and apply Sunflower Shea Summer Oil (page 158). Your skin will feel and look glowy and smooth!

MAKES 8 OUNCES

1 cup coconut sugar

1 tablespoon maca root powder

2 tablespoons sunflower oil

3 drops holy basil essential oil

In a bowl, whisk together the sugar and maca powder until fully blended. Maca has a tendency to stay clumped, so be sure to break down the clumps prior to adding the oils. Add the sunflower oil and holy basil essential oil, and continue to whisk until all the ingredients are fully blended. Store in an airtight container at room temperature. Use within 7 days.

pomegranate and melissa oil dense fall scrub

THIS SCRUB COUNTERACTS THE ANXIETY THAT CAN ACCOMPANY FALL BY WRAPPING *us up in a comforting blanket of sesame oil, bolstered by the strengthening properties of pomegranate, plus Melissa (lemon balm) essential oil to soothe and calm your central nervous system. This scrub's texture is denser than the others. Sesame oil is used often in Ayurveda because it is so rich in vitamins and minerals. Your skin will thank you!*

You can apply this scrub in the shower, with the water on, gliding it all over your body, exfoliating and then massaging the oil deeply into your tissues as the sugar crystals dissolve. After you are done in the shower, pat your body dry with a towel. A nice layer of the oil will remain on your skin. Feel free to apply more Orange Sesame Fall Oil (page 158) if you are feeling extra-sensitive or are experiencing higher levels of anxiety.

MAKES 8 OUNCES

1 cup coconut sugar

2 tablespoons pomegranate powder

8 to 10 tablespoons sesame oil

10 to 12 drops Melissa essential oil

In a bowl, whisk together the sugar and powder until they are fully blended. Add the sesame oil and Melissa essential oil and continue to blend until all the ingredients are combined. Store in an airtight container at room temperature. Use within 7 days.

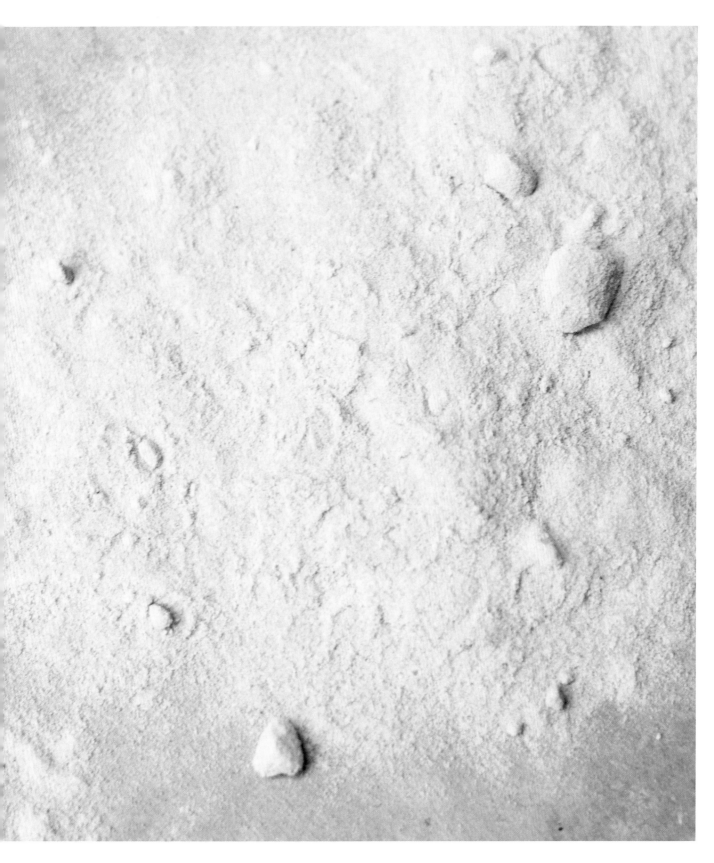

seasonal body oils

I love oils and use them every day, all over my body and on my face, too. Each type of oil has its own set of characteristics and nourishing benefits, and when blended together, they become a rich and enriching tonic for the skin.

All of the oils in these blends have been carefully selected to deliver specific nourishing benefits to your skin for each season, to help you maintain a healthy glow and feel more balanced, alive, and awakened. You can blend these oils in an ordinary kitchen measuring cup, which I often do, or you can use laboratory beakers. The oils should be stored in a darkened glass container. I prefer 100 ml Infinity Jars. If you do the daily self-massage, the 4-ounce yield of these recipes should last for approximately one week.

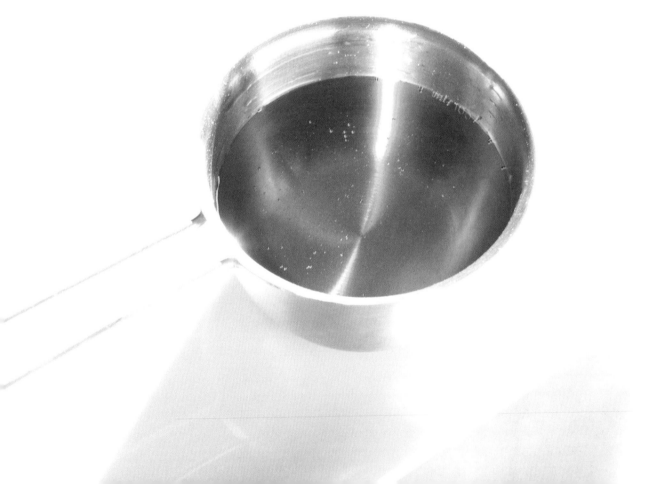

grapefruit avocado winter oil

THE COMBINATION OF OLIVE AND AVOCADO OIL WILL WARD OFF THOSE DRY SKIN *winter blues. The fatty acid content of olive oil is just what your dry skin needs, while the grapefruit essential oil is anti-inflammatory. Avocado will ensure that all of this goodness penetrates and softens your skin. The chamomile essential oil is a nervine and smooths out overall stressors to the mind, body, and spirit.*

MAKES 4 OUNCES

¼ cup extra-virgin olive oil

¼ cup avocado oil

3 to 4 drops grapefruit essential oil

2 drops chamomile essential oil

Pour the olive and avocado oil into a glass measuring cup or beaker and stir them together. Add the grapefruit and chamomile essential oils and stir some more. Transfer the oil to a dark glass storage container. Use approximately 1 tablespoon per day for your self-massage.

lemon primrose spring oil

PRIMROSE IS LIKE A DREAM. IT'S RICH IN OMEGA-6 FATTY ACIDS, SOOTHES THE SKIN, *and has the magical ability to smooth out wrinkles. Rose hip oil is a natural source of vitamin A, with a retinol effect that boosts collagen and increases cellular turnover. Lemon essential oil purifies the skin and energizes.*

MAKES 4 OUNCES

¼ cup evening primrose oil

¼ cup rose hips oil

4 to 5 drops lemon essential oil

Pour the primrose and rose hips into a glass measuring cup or beaker and stir them together. Add the lemon essential oils and stir all the ingredients together. Transfer the oil to a storage container. Use approximately 1 tablespoon per day for your self-massage.

sunflower shea summer oil

SHEA OIL MAKES A GREAT SUMMER BASE BECAUSE IT'S LIGHT AND ABSORBS QUICKLY. *Not only that, but it's extremely moisturizing and rich in vitamin E. Sunflower oil promotes hydration, while holy basil essential oil increases endurance and relieves joint pain.*

MAKES 4 OUNCES

¼ cup shea oil

¼ cup sunflower oil

3 to 4 drops holy basil essential oil

Pour the shea and sunflower oils into a glass measuring cup or beaker and stir them together. Add the holy basil essential oil and stir until all the ingredients are combined. Transfer to a storage container. Use approximately 1 tablespoon per day for your self-massage.

orange sesame fall oil

SESAME OIL IS USED OFTEN IN AYURVEDA BECAUSE IT IS SO RICH IN VITAMINS *and minerals. Fig seed oil is high in vitamin A, which stimulates collagen production, and vitamin K, which promotes skin elasticity. Orange essential oil boosts immunity, alleviates depression, and is an anti-inflammatory.*

MAKES 4 OUNCES

¼ cup sesame oil

¼ cup fig seed or prickly pear oil

5 to 7 drops orange essential oil

Pour the sesame and fig seed oils into a glass measuring cup or beaker and stir them together. Add the orange essential oil and stir some more. Transfer the oil to a storage container. Use approximately 1 tablespoon per day for your self-massage.

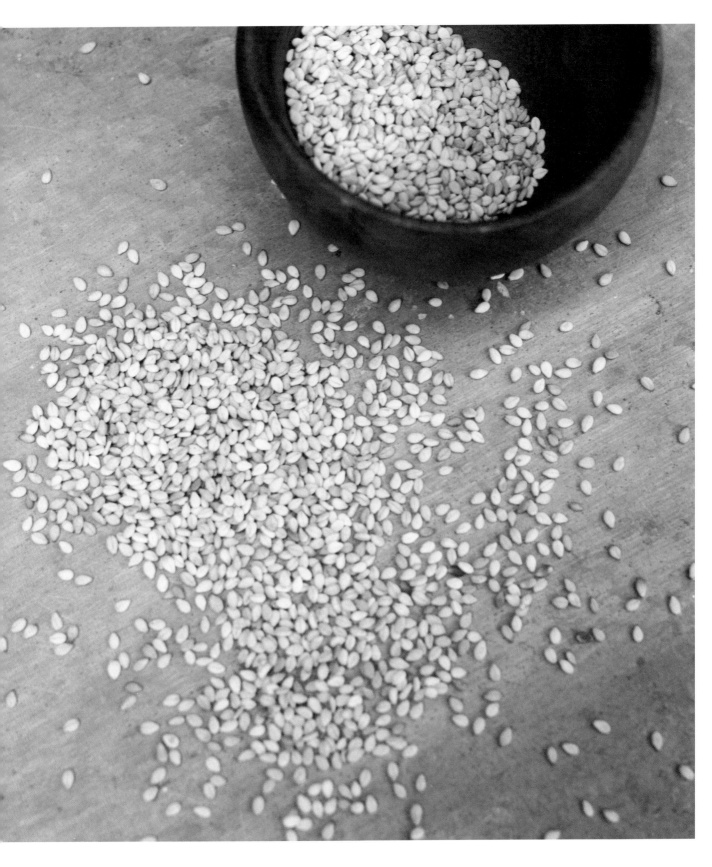

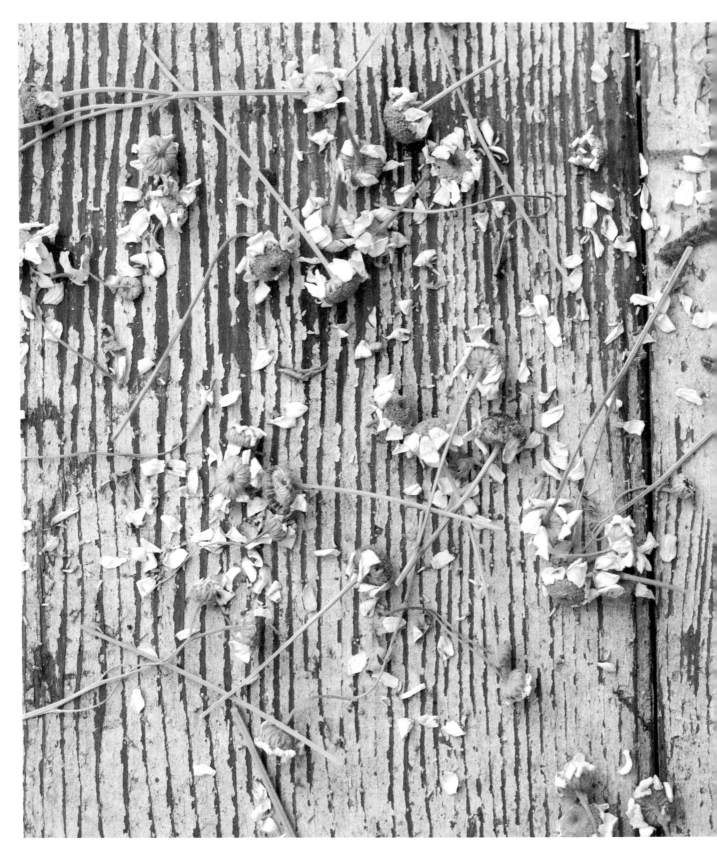

seasonal mists

I use mists to spritz my face for some extra glow, as well as for a pick-me-up during the day. I also like to spray them around my environment to add a delicious scent. Their presence clears my mind and perks my senses. I've added essential oils as well as some fresh ingredients to provide more depth and whole plant medicine. All of these mists are packed with powerful vitamins and minerals to benefit the skin.

grapefruit chamomile winter mist

GRAPEFRUIT STIMULATES THE IMMUNE SYSTEM, CURBS SUGAR CRAVINGS, AND *alleviates symptoms of depression. Chamomile is calming, relieves anxiety, and helps alleviate insomnia.*

MAKES 4 OUNCES

1 grapefruit wedge

½ cup distilled water

½ teaspoon vegetable glycerin

2 drops chamomile essential oil

2 drops grapefruit essential oil

Squeeze the grapefruit wedge into a container and remove the seeds to create grapefruit juice. In a glass measuring cup or beaker, mix together 1 teaspoon of this grapefruit juice and the water, glycerin, and chamomile and grapefruit essential oils. Transfer the mist to a container (preferably glass) with a spritzer cap and refrigerate. This mist should last for 2 to 3 days.

jasmine lemon spring mist

JASMINE AND LEMON ARE SUCH A YUMMY BLEND FOR SPRING! JASMINE HAS A *delightful effect on the mind and uplifts the mood, while lemon energizes and purifies the skin.*

MAKES 4 OUNCES

1 lemon wedge

½ cup distilled water

½ teaspoon vegetable glycerin

1 drop jasmine essential oil

1 drop lemon essential oil

Squeeze the lemon wedge into a container and remove the seeds. In a glass measuring cup or container, mix together 1 teaspoon of the lemon juice and the water, glycerin, jasmine essential oil, and lemon essential oil. Transfer the mist to a container (preferably glass) with a spritzer cap and refrigerate. The mist should last for 2 to 3 days.

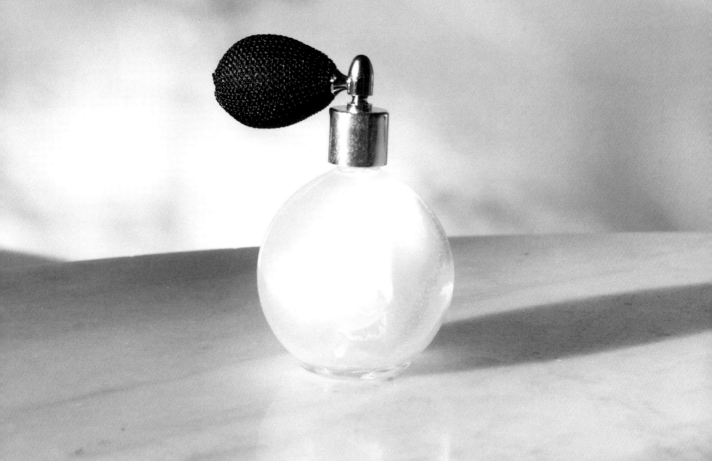

basil cucumber summer mist

LIME JUICE BRIGHTENS SKIN, WHILE CUCUMBER DIMINISHES SWELLING AND *puffiness, especially around the eyes. Basil heals and smooths out feelings of stress and anxiety.*

MAKES 4 OUNCES

1 lime wedge

1 small cucumber

½ cup distilled water

½ teaspoon vegetable glycerin

1 drop basil essential oil

Squeeze the lime wedge into a container and remove the seeds. Juice the cucumber in a juicer. In a glass measuring cup or container, mix together 1 teaspoon of the lime juice, 2 tablespoons of the cucumber juice, and the water, glycerin, and basil essential oil. Transfer the mist to a container (preferably glass) with a spritzer cap and refrigerate. The mist should last for 2 to 3 days.

Be sure to drink the leftover cucumber juice, as it contains high amounts of stress-reducing magnesium!

orange ginger fall mist

BOOST YOUR IMMUNE SYSTEM, REDUCE INFLAMMATION, AND IMPROVE THE OVERALL *health of your skin inside and out with this warming mist.*

MAKES 4 OUNCES

1 (1-inch) piece fresh ginger

1 orange wedge

½ cup distilled water

½ teaspoon vegetable glycerin

1 to 2 drops orange essential oil

Juice the ginger and the orange wedge separately, reserving 2 drops of ginger and 1 teaspoon of orange juice. Combine the remaining orange and ginger juice and drink them up! In a glass measuring cup or container, mix together the 2 drops of ginger juice, 1 teaspoon of orange juice, and water, glycerin, and orange essential oil. Transfer the mist to a container (preferably glass) with a spritzer cap and refrigerate. The mist should last for 2 to 3 days.

seasonal soaks

Seasonal soaks are profoundly healing. Hot water opens our pores and causes us to sweat, which detoxifies the body, as well as the mind and spirit. These soaks are incredibly simple to make and are prepared directly into a freshly drawn bath.

Begin by setting a relaxing mood for yourself. Dim the lights and add some candles for ambience, play some relaxing music, a spoken meditation, or maybe even a recording of poetry.

Run the water to a temperature of your liking. As the water is running, evenly disperse an 8-pound bag of magnesium chloride flakes (I like the Ancient Minerals brand). These flakes are great for a host of issues, including reducing symptoms of fatigue, insomnia, and chronic pain; relieving mental and physical tension; as well as alleviating skin conditions, such as psoriasis and eczema. I use the entire contents of an 8-pound bag per bath to maximize the benefits of the magnesium.

I use magnesium chloride flakes all year long, and an essential oil specific to a season:

Winter: 3 to 4 drops of lemongrass essential oil

Spring: 3 to 4 drops of rose essential oil

Summer: 3 to 4 drops of holy basil essential oil

Fall: 3 to 4 drops of orange essential oil

After you've added the essential oil, swish your hand through the water to further disperse the oils. Soak for 20 to 30 minutes. During the winter and fall seasons, you can use the seasonal scrub on your body while lying in the bath; in the spring and summer months you can use the dry exfoliating powder prior to immersing yourself in the bath.

When you finish the bath, pat yourself dry with a towel and apply the appropriate seasonal oil to lock in moisture, spritz your face with a seasonal mist, and receive a powerful combination of nourishing benefits to your skin, mind, and spirit.

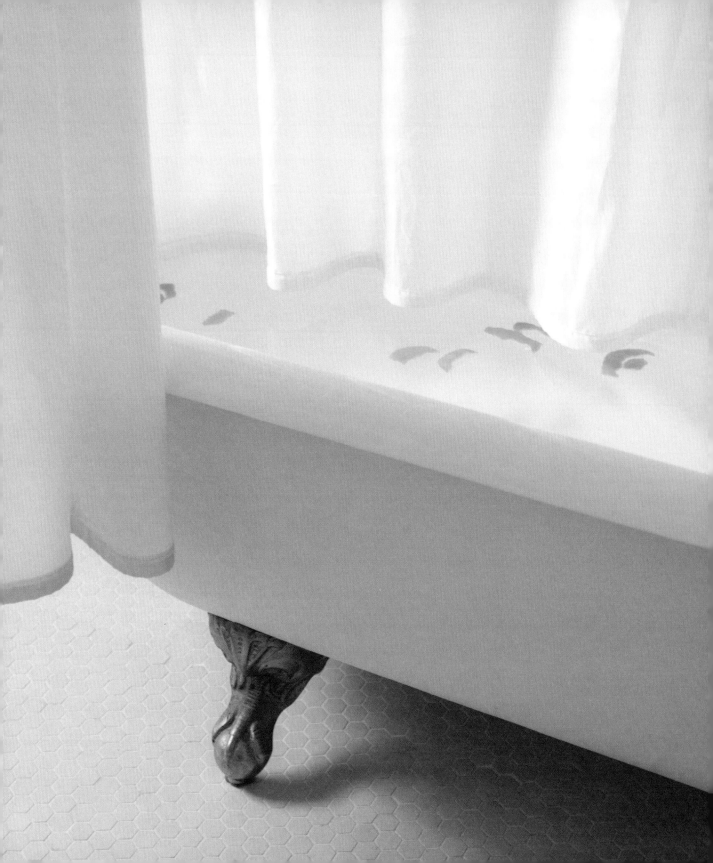

think and meditate: savor the silence

The entire Slow Beauty practice is a form of meditation. It is in the silent moments, the emptiness, when deep renewal occurs. Silence *is* a sound, and it is the most beautiful sound to behold. Now, if only we heard that gorgeous sound more often!

Perhaps it initially seems a bit weird to put "thinking" and "meditating" together in a single section. After all, we're frequently told that meditation is all about shutting off our brain and clearing our thoughts. Nope—impossible. In fact, it is all but certain that at some point in your meditation practice, uncomfortable thoughts will pop into your head, and you will need to sit with them—to share the silence with them. This is a way to cultivate bravery. Meditation is *not* about stopping your thoughts; instead, it's about creating space between you and your thoughts so you don't do what I like to call "thought-clinging." Of course, there are some thoughts we want to hold on to, like when we are trying to find a solution to a problem, and then there are others types of "thought forms" that we cling to that are not beneficial to us. They are thoughts that will bring us down or make us feel heavy, and will wreak havoc on our

central nervous system. They have the potential to take over if we entertain them for too long. Those are the thoughts I'm talking about, those are the thoughts you will need to watch come and go—especially go. *Sayonara!*

Incorporating a meditation practice into our life is unspeakably powerful. In the eighteen years since I have been meditating, I've found that my meditation practice has come to the rescue many times over. When I sit down to meditate, I feel stress melting away, which is especially beneficial during flu and cold season, when stress contributes to the weakening of our immune system. It also helps smooth things over when something external has pushed a button that triggers a flow of unsavory thoughts.

In addition to meditation, we will also incorporate such practices as breathing, visualization, and mantras. All of these nicely supplement meditation by slowing us down and giving us a point of focus. However, they can be done completely on their own to great benefit.

mantras

One of my favorite ways to change my mind-set and outlook is through mantras. A mantra is an intentional word, sound, or phrase that assists us in a mindfulness practice like meditation. The yogi guru B. K. S. Iyengar explained mantras as a "sacred thought or prayer" meant to be repeated. In fact, mantras are so powerful that they are considered to be one of the paths to enlightenment in the yogic tradition. Because mantras are so sacred and powerful, it's important that we choose our own mantras thoughtfully, and that they resonate deep within us. It is a guide that assists us in deep relaxation. It is a tool that helps detoxify the mind, body, and spirit of negative and unsupportive thinking and behavior.

Traditionally, teachers assign mantras to their students, selecting phrases they believe will assist the student in his or her personal growth. Whether we are designing our own mantras or they are passed along to us, a mantra is ultimately a tool to help us develop an inner life that is most aligned with our personal values and authentic self. There are lifelong mantras, and there are also shorter-term ones meant to accompany us through specific phases of our life.

There are many ways to receive and use a mantra. I personally practice a form of meditation known as Transcendental Meditation. As part of the learning process, each student is given a mantra in the form of a sound. This mantra is passed along from teacher to student by being said aloud once by the teacher when the mantra is "assigned," and once by the student when he or she "receives" it. After this, the mantra is repeated over and over again, but only silently as the student practices two twenty-minute meditations per day, using the mantra as a focal point. The mantra is considered so sacred and personally meaningful that it is never to be shared with anyone other than the student and teacher.

create your own mantra

Now, having said all of that, the only guru or teacher you actually need to lead you through your own mantra and/or meditation practice is *you*. You *are* your own guru because, after all, who knows you and your innermost desires better than yourself?

As you begin to turn your mind toward creating your very own mantra, allow yourself to slow down and engage in the very highest form of knowledge: your intuition. Each of us is the keeper of both our questions *and* our answers. One of the best ways to allow for this slowing down and engagement is through meditation or practices in mindfulness (such as yoga, mindful walking, swimming, or whatever mode you may use to engage body, mind, and spirit and delve within).

If you don't already have a meditation or mindfulness practice, here are a few tips for slowing things down to obtain the clarity of mind necessary to design a mantra that will resonate with you. The point of this exercise is to bring yourself into a state of calm that allows you to create an internal space where expansive thoughts can arise. When you've found that calm, creative space where all of the outside noise from day-to-day life fades away, notice what happens. Are there any words, phrases, or sounds that come up and resonate with you? Anything that makes you feel especially good or joyful or safe? It doesn't have to be complicated—and it doesn't even necessarily have to make sense in the context of the logical mind. You're allowing what is on the inside to rise up to the surface, and sometimes we are surprised by what we find there. Whatever it is you find that speaks to you, *that* will be your mantra.

Now, I understand that, based on the popular understanding of meditation, it may seem counter-intuitive to specifically create or invite thoughts when we are meditating, which is, indeed, what we're doing when seeking out our own mantra. But, remember, first of all, there are many different kinds of meditation. Second, and most important, even when we meditate, we are still *human*. And humans have thoughts. As we've already touched on, the point is not to turn our mind into a completely blank slate—that would be impossible. The point is to "de-clutter" our mind so that we can become more in touch with who we really are in the deepest part of ourself and what we believe in the most and hold the most dear. Thoughts come and go. In meditation, we want to allow them to come and go without judging them and qualifying them as "good" or "bad." It is in this place that you will find your mantra.

To get started:

1. Find a quiet, comfortable place to sit—somewhere you will not be interrupted for at least fifteen minutes. This may sound like a lot of time if you are new to meditation, but I promise that you'll soon come to cherish this part of the day that's just for you. You may want to consider downloading an app, such as Insight Timer or Meditation Timer, to track your time for you. Be sure that you have nearby a journal or something to write in.

2. Sit down on a chair or stool, place your feet on the ground, and let your hands rest gently on your lap, palms facing either up or down. Take care not to cross anything—you want your feet to be grounded to the earth and your heart to be open. Let your eyes gently close.

③ Take three rounds of deep and full inhalations and exhalations through your nose, feeling the incoming air travel all the way down to your diaphragm and releasing all the air back out on the exhale. As you inhale, envision yourself breathing in *calm*; as you exhale, breathe out *stress*.

④ Repeat the breathing process, this time both inhaling and exhaling calm.

Continue this process of full, deep breathing. As you do, direct your mind's eye toward the positive image you'd like to set for your conceptualization of beauty. As you breathe, allow your thoughts to arise naturally. Let them come, and let them go. Remain here for the duration of the fifteen-minute meditation (or for as long as you would like to sit).

⑤ Immediately after you've finished your meditation, record any thoughts that arose in your journal. It is from this exercise that we will allow ourself to find our own answers and determine our mantra from there. You may have your mantra after one meditation session, or it may take you a few. Be patient with the process.

Once you have identified your mantra, emblazon it on your heart, keep it to yourself, and profess it to yourself internally. This is *your* mantra. It came *to* you and *from* you. Use it anytime and anywhere you please, whether it's the focus of a formal meditation or mindfulness session, as a quick reminder, or whenever you need a shot of good vibrations. I find it helpful to connect with my mantra first thing in the morning, as a way of focusing and starting my day off on the right note. Some people like to use it at some point during the day to check in and, if necessary, recalibrate—or to just keep moving along that beautiful, positive path. Should negative thinking or self-talk arise, that is the perfect time to use your mantra to shift your thinking to a more positive state.

Whatever feels most comfortable and natural to you is the exact way you should use your mantra. The more regularly you use your mantra, the more effective, transformative, and powerful it will be.

breathe: connect deeply with life

I often find myself breathing shallowly in those moments when I'm under a lot of stress. At times, this becomes so extreme that I'm all but holding my breath. Ironically for me—and probably for you, too—I tend to hold my breath during those moments when I need it the most. Breathing brings us into the moment. It calms us. It slows us down. It regulates our nervous system and attunes us with our own body. And, in addition to all of this, breathing can be extremely meditative.

The purpose of *pranayama* (Sanskrit for "breath") is to direct energy into the spine and brain. Breath focuses the energy in the power line of our body; it redirects it from being expended and wasted on external nonsense, such as stress. In short, it sets us straight. Along with yoga and meditation, breathwork has gained popularity and recognition in recent years. Still, its power to transform is largely underestimated. If we are what we eat and what we think, we are even more so how we breathe. When we breathe deeply and fluidly, our experience of life will also be more deep and fluid.

As with the more traditional recipes earlier in this part of the book, I will also provide *pranayama* (another word for breathwork) "recipes"

for each season. These various techniques will provide you with a means of accessing energy that is dormant or stuck within your body, as well as with the energy you need for a particular season. As with nutrition, also with breath: Each season requires a unique breathing technique to tap into what your mind, body, and spirit require during that particular cycle.

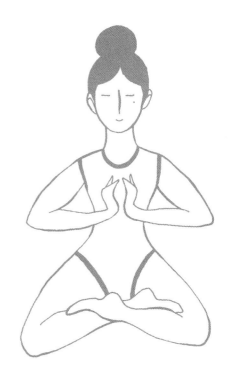

heat-generating winter breath

This breathing technique uses the right nostril to generate heat in the body. It's a great exercise for winter, when we need to generate a bit of extra heat from the inside out. This breathing technique increases energy and vitality, improves digestion, and reduces anxiety and depression. Note: Do not complete this exercise if you have high blood pressure.

Begin by sitting in a comfortable cross-legged position, with your spine erect. Place your right elbow on your left palm. Using your ring finger, close your left nostril. Inhale through your right nostril as you slowly count to four, remove your finger from your left nostril, and exhale through your left nostril as you count to four. Repeat this breathing pattern ten times. As you continue practicing and build up more stamina, work your way up to eighty breaths total. Eventually your exhale should be double the amount of your inhale. When you are done, take a few moments to breathe in and out through both nostrils before you go about your daily activities.

bhramari spring breath

Bhramari means "bee" in Sanskrit, and this exercise is so named because of the humming sound it creates in the back of the throat. I like to use this breath in the spring because this season is a time of fertilization, which always makes me think of our bumblebee friends. This powerful form of breathing reduces fatigue and mental stress; reduces anxiety, frustration, and anger; and improves concentration. Not only that, but it also positively impacts ear, nose, mouth, and eye issues, and since spring is the season when we are prone to more allergies, we really want to keep these areas healthy. This simple breathing technique can be practiced anywhere, which makes it a great option for on-the-spot de-stressing.

Sit comfortably in a chair or on the floor, with your spine straight. Close your eyes and bring your attention to your breath. Listen to all of the sounds around you, starting with the ones far away, moving in to the ones closest to you, inhaling deeply and exhaling deeply. Once you have come into a regular, steady breath pattern, lift your index fingers to your ears, and gently press on the tragus (the small cartilage part of your ear), gently closing them (do not put your fingers inside your ear). Keeping your mouth closed, slowly inhale through your nostrils and on the exhale make a high-pitched humming sound like a bee as you release your breath through your nose. Pause at the bottom of your breath, then inhale slowly and fully. Repeat this cycle five times.

cooling summer breath

Just as we can use our breath to warm up in the winter, in the summer we can use it to cool down. This is a great breathing technique for summer when we are feeling a bit overwhelmed from the intense summer heat. Breathing through your left nostril soothes emotions, is calming, cooling, and helps when you can't get to sleep.

Sit in a comfortable position and align your head, neck, and spine. Start to pay attention to your breathing; after a few breaths, close your eyes to go deeper with your concentration. Breathe in and out naturally, feeling your breath travel throughout your body on the inhale. On the exhale, release the breath from your body.

Once you feel connected with your breath, open your mouth and curl your tongue length-wise, then stick out your tongue. Pretend you are drinking through a straw as you inhale across your tongue and into your mouth. Notice the cooling sensation of your breath. Bring your tongue back in, close your mouth, and exhale completely through your nostrils.

Repeat this breathing pattern for two to three minutes to start, ultimately working your way up to ten minutes.

IF YOU CAN'T CURL YOUR TONGUE

If curling your tongue isn't an option for Cooling Summer Breath, instead gently press your lower and upper teeth together and separate your lips as much as you comfortably can, exposing your teeth to the air. Inhale slowly through your teeth, focusing on the hissing sound of the breath. Close your mouth and slowly exhale through the nose.

This breathing technique offers all of the same cooling effects as Cooling Summer Breath, *plus* it balances the endocrine system and builds vitality.

tonglen fall breath

During the fall season we are more prone to worry and feelings of anxiety, which wreak havoc on our central nervous system. When this occurs, tonglen is the perfect breathing exercise to help bring us back to a balanced state. With this breath, we will transform our burdened state of mind to one that is more elevated and expanded, freeing ourself from those things that are keeping us imprisoned in a depressed state of being. Through this breathwork, we are being radically inclusive about those aspects of ourself that we would rather ostracize and push out to the margins. We are going to sit with these feelings, and transform them. The purpose of tonglen is to help us be more compassionate with ourself and, from there, to be more compassionate with others. When someone shows up in our life who is "breathing out" something difficult, we will now have the tools to be inclusive and help transform those "vibes" so they don't weigh us down.

Sit comfortably in a chair with your feet on the ground and your hands placed gently on your lap, breathing easily. Focus on your breath, making your inhales and exhales longer and deeper for about three rounds of breath. Now, on your next inhale, breathe in the uncomfortable feeling that has you imprisoned. I know it sounds counterintuitive, but you are going to bring near what is making you feel uncomfortable. On the exhale, breathe out its opposite, the feeling that makes you feel elevated, expansive, and at your best. Continue breathing in this way for seven to ten more rounds.

move: use energy to stir your soul

You can think of movement as a full-body prayer. Praying is an act of connecting with the divine, which includes your divine self. What better way to connect with ourself and our divinity than through our body? We can move in gratitude, we can move as a form of expression, we can move to de-stress, and to energize.

There is also a far more practical component to movement, which is that, bottom line: Movement is a vital component of good health. Part of this 24/7 lifestyle we live today demands that we spend so much time sitting. *Too* much time sitting. We sit at our jobs, sometimes for hours at a time. We are glued to our computers, smartphones, and tablets, all of which takes a toll on our body.

Remember that movement is the body's language. We are born to move. As children, we are incredibly active—we have so much energy, which courses through our body and expresses itself in spontaneous movement. But as soon as school begins, we are told to sit still and be quiet. Over time, we lose touch with our body's natural and spontaneous expressions. Movement becomes available only to those who show talent, and who are deemed worthy.

I'm here to tell you that you don't need to be a trained movement artist to enjoy the language of the body. The movement recipes in this section are designed to awaken and help you get back in touch with this language within you. I am not a technically trained dancer or yoga instructor. My "training" amounts to hours upon hours of creating dance routines in front of the mirrored closets in the foyer of my childhood home and, later on, years of yoga classes. I just love to dance and move my body. I love dance so much I wish life were a music video and we could all just dance through it. As you incorporate the movements in this section into your own Slow Beauty practice, please remember that perfection is not the goal. What we are going for here is creating space for

ourself and our own unique expression. When we move our body, we are having a conversation with ourself and with the world. We are saying things like "I am open," "I am flexible," "I am fluid," "I am joyful," and "I am creative." We are expressing so many beautiful messages to every cell in our body. We are energizing ourself and creating reserves of energy to use throughout our day.

winter movements: invigorate and calm

Belly Dancing

Belly dancing is a great way to build core strength and stability, boost our immunity, reduce stress and tension, boost self-confidence, improve circulation and suppleness, increase joint flexibility, deepen our breath, and tone all major muscle groups.

HIP ISOLATIONS

Begin with your legs lined up under your hip-bones, knees slightly bent, abs tucked, chest lifted, and arms out. Maintaining this posture, bend your knees a bit more. Now, straighten your right knee so that the right hip shifts up, and then bend your right knee again to re-center your hips. Repeat this same movement on the left side, straightening your left knee so that the left hip shifts up, then bending your left knee again to re-center your hips. As you move, keep your heels planted on the floor. This will make it easier to find these isolated movements.

Continue to move in this manner, for a total of fifty isolations on each side, switching from side to side.

ARM MOVEMENTS

Once you're comfortable with hip isolations, we'll start to incorporate arm movements. When we're belly dancing, our arms always remain energetic. Relax your shoulders and position your arms in start position as if you are holding a large beach ball. Now open and close your arms as if you were expanding the size of the ball, moving your wrists backward and forward.

TEMPLE ARMS

Alternatively, we can use Temple Arms. In this position, lift your arms above your head, keeping your shoulders drawn down. Cross your wrists over your head, drawing your elbows back. From this position, allow your hands to move, using them as a form of expression. Have fun with this!

Warrior Series

Yoga builds strength, flexibility, and balance, both physically and mentally. It's also a great practice for fusing together movement and breathwork. The more we practice this on the mat, the more we'll find ourself breathing fully and deeply in our day-to-day life as well.

WARRIOR 1

Start out by standing with your feet hips' width apart at the top of your mat. From there, step your left foot back about 3 feet. Bend your right knee as close to 90 degrees as possible, trying to get your right thigh parallel to the mat. Turn your left foot out slightly at a 45-degree angle, so that your toes are pointed toward the top left corner of your yoga mat. Staying strong in your stance, on an inhale, lift your arms up toward the sky, palms facing in toward each other, as you continue to draw your shoulder blades down to maintain a long neck. Continue breathing for five long, fluid breaths as you hold this pose. As you settle into the posture, see whether you can point your tailbone down toward the mat a little more, keeping your abs firm and strong.

WARRIOR 2

At the top of your sixth exhale, we will shift into Warrior 2. As you inhale, windmill your arms and pivot your body so that your arms are in a T shape, right arm pointed in front of you, left arm behind you. Adjust your feet slightly so that the back of your right heel bisects the arch of your left foot. Draw your shoulders down, finding that long neck once again. Make sure you are maintaining that 90-degree bend in your front knee, and that your right knee is not collapsing in toward the left. Your torso should be positioned directly above your hips so that your chest is facing the wall to your left. Hold this pose for five more deep breaths, continuing to ground your feet down for a solid foundation, while keeping your upper body as light as possible. At the end of your fifth exhale, gently step your left foot up to join your right and return to your beginning position at the top of the mat. Repeat on the other side, again for five full breaths on each side.

Ballet

Ballet is so elegant, so graceful. Chances are you took at least a class or two when you were a little girl. Time to get back in touch with those days. Ballet is all about grace, fluidity, and strength. Positions one through five are easy to do and have great benefits to the body, like improving posture, strengthening the inner core, and toning the arms and thighs.

To enjoy the fluidity of these movements, each position should flow into the one that follows. Try ten sets in sequence, moving from first position through fifth position.

1ST POSITION

Stand with your heels together, toes apart, comfortable and balanced. Relax your hands and place them in front of your thighs (but not quite touching them), apart by approximately the width of your face, as if you were holding a beach ball.

2ND POSITION

With a sliding motion, move one foot the length of your foot and a half apart from the other foot. Raise your arms in a smooth transition from first position, until they are almost at the height of your shoulders. Then open them up into a straight line at your sides with your hands relaxed.

3RD POSITION

Slide the heel of your foot and place it in front of the arch of your back foot. Leave one arm in second position and bring the other arm in front of you.

4TH POSITION

Slide your front foot approximately one foot size in front of you. Raise the arm that is opposite the foot and keep your other arm in second position.

5TH POSITION

Slide the heel of your front foot toward the big toe of your back foot and place it in front of the big toe. Raise your other arm above your head so that both arms are lifted, elbows and arms relaxed, not pointing but not drooping, either.

spring movements: expand

Meandering Movement

This spontaneous movement exercise will help you get in touch with how your body naturally moves. It will help you get "unstuck" physically, mentally, and emotionally. Although you may do this exercise at any time of the day—and multiple times a day, for that matter—I especially like doing it first thing in the morning (kind of like "morning pages" from Julia Cameron's *The Artist's Way*), and anytime during the day when you feel stagnant.

When you wake up and dance first thing in the morning, notice how your day begins. This is a dance diary that exists only in the moment, and then it is gone. You write it from a clean slate each day and your body won't move the same way all the time; in fact, it will move differently every day.

To start your day with this movement, sit up in bed without first touching your cell phone; in fact, make sure your cell phone isn't even in your bedroom. Place your feet on the floor and then start to move your body. If you are on your way to the bathroom, dance. This dance might be a slow meandering walk with spontaneous outbursts of your arms or anything else that moves you. There is no right or wrong way to do this, you just need to let your body express itself. If you feel sluggish, then move in a sluggish way; if you feel buoyant, then bounce your way to where you are headed; if you are reenacting a dream from the previous night, do whatever that entails.

Although your dance exists only in the moment, your body will remember it. It will have an impact on you; you don't have to write about it or photograph it. The point is to not trap your movement, pin it down, document it, own it, or objectify it. It's to set the movement free, like a yawn or a sneeze. It lasts for a brief moment, and then it is gone.

Tapping

Tapping, which is used as a form of holistic medicine to unlock energy, is a great way to increase vitality and energy. Stand up and, using the tips of your fingers, start under your eyes and gently tap, moving back and forth on the skin under your eyes, for approximately thirty seconds. Next, move to your collarbones and use your opposite hand to tap on your collarbone area with a bit more vigor. Move to your thymus (center of chest above breastbones) and, using either hand, tap with the same pressure you used on your collarbone for thirty seconds. Finally, move to your spleen, the largest lymphatic system in the body, and tap with your right hand for thirty seconds.

Breath of Joy

This is a breathing exercise, but it is also movement in the Kripalu yoga tradition. I love this practice because it awakens the entire system as it moves energy throughout the body, uplifting mind, body, and spirit, and promoting a sense of calm and focus.

To begin, stand with your feet shoulders' width apart and knees slightly bent. Inhale partially and then swing your arms in front of your body, then over your head, making sure they are parallel to each other at shoulder level with the palms facing each other. Inhale more as you stretch your arms out to your sides at shoulder height, opening them as if they were your wings. Inhale to full lung capacity, swinging your arms back to parallel over your head with palms facing each other.

Open your mouth, letting out a loud and clear "*haaa*" as you exhale, as you bend your knees to sink into a standing squat, and swing your arms down and back behind you like a diver. Repeat this breath and movement cycle up to ten times. Enjoy the flow of the rhythm of this technique.

Once you have completed your final round, return to standing position and close your eyes. Notice the effect this movement has had on your body, paying special attention to your beating heart, and the other tingling sensations throughout your body. Notice how alive you are, and how joyful that is.

summer movements: moderate

Moon Salutation

This yoga sequence is a full-body prayer, which can be a particularly poignant exercise when done on the new and full moon as we alternately set our intentions and acknowledge the completion of cycles. It is a cooling flow of movement, which is perfect for the summer months.

Begin by standing at the top of your mat, feet hips' width distance apart. As you inhale, lift your arms up over your head, palms facing in toward each other, shoulder blades drawn down. On the exhale, fold forward, maintaining a flat back and leading with your heart as you crease at the hips. Inhale and, keeping your feet where they are, lower your bottom so that you are in a squat. Exhale, and step your left leg back so that you are in a low lunge, left knee on the mat. Inhale, and lift your arms up overhead, palms facing in. Exhale, bring your hands down to the mat to frame your feet. As you inhale, step your back leg forward and bring both knees to the mat so that you are sitting up on your knees in Hero Pose. Exhale, then inhale again as you lift your arms toward the sky, taking a slight backbend if it feels good. Exhale, sit your hips back on your feet, release your arms forward and find Child's Pose. Stay here for a round of breath or two.

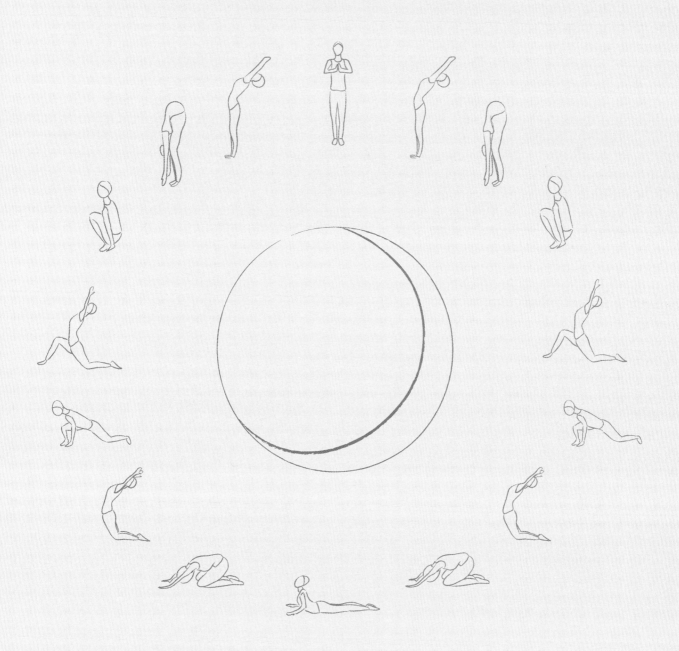

On an inhale, staying low to the mat, draw your torso forward. Place your hands directly under your shoulders, draw your shoulders down and back and, keeping a bend in your elbows, lift your chest to come into Cobra Pose. As you exhale, release back to Child's Pose. Inhale, lift up on your knees, lifting your arms above your head, returning to Hero Pose.

Exhale, step your right leg back into a low lunge, hands framing the front foot. Inhale, lift your torso and raise your arms over your head. Exhale, step your right leg forward to meet your left, coming into a squat. Inhale, as you begin to straighten your legs to lift and exhale, release yourself into a forward fold. Inhale, rise up from your hip crease with a flat back, lifting your arms overhead, and exhale, release your arms through your center, bringing them into prayer at your heart.

Repeat this flow for as many rounds as you would like, allowing yourself to sink into a flowing rhythm of movement and breath.

Seated Forward Fold

This static movement is a great release for the back, hamstrings, and your distracted mind.

Sit on your mat with your legs stretched in front of you. Throughout this movement, allow your knees to be as bent as necessary, depending on how tight your hamstrings are, but be sure to leave at least a microbend to protect the knees.

As you inhale, lift your arms up overhead. Exhale, crease at the hips, maintain a straight spine as you release forward. Don't push anything and take this movement measure by measure. Each time you breathe in, see whether you can lengthen by straightening your spine a bit. Each time you exhale, see whether you can let go and release a bit more, drawing your torso a bit closer to your knees. Never push yourself in a forward fold—this is all about micromovements and not pushing yourself too far. After about five rounds of breath, on the sixth exhale, allow your spine to release and relax as you release any tension in your torso, letting yourself fold forward. Allow your breath to return to a normal, uncontrolled pattern as you let go in the fold.

When you are ready to come out on an inhale, slowly draw yourself up and return to a seated position.

Standing Forward Fold

Much like Seated Forward Fold, Standing Forward Fold is a great pose for down-cycling and releasing the hamstrings. It also lengthens the inner legs, reduces stress and tension in the head and neck, calms the mind, and alleviates fatigue.

Begin with your feet planted on the mat, hips' width apart, keeping at least a slight bend in the knee. Inhale as you lift your arms up overhead and exhale, crease at the hips to fold forward. From the folded position, allow your torso to be heavy and relax your neck. See whether you can lift your sit bones up toward the sky. With each inhale, think about lifting and lengthening the body; with each exhale, allow yourself to grow heavy and fold a little deeper. Maybe allow your torso to sway slightly from side to side, nod your head yes, and shake it no.

When you are ready, on an inhale, roll yourself up one vertebra at a time, keeping your head heavy and allowing it to be the last part of you to lift.

fall movements: let go

Miming

Yes, you read that right. We are going to use miming as a form of movement. You're most welcome to dust off your bowler hat, but it's not necessary. Miming may seem like an antiquated art, but even the late, great David Bowie was inspired by mimes. And it doesn't get much cooler than Bowie. In case you don't know, mimes are silent storytellers who use their body and facial expressions in lieu of their voice. Miming is also a wonderful way to tap into our imagination, creativity, and humor.

Fall can be a pretty windy time of year, and in the Ayurvedic tradition, it is associated with a lack of groundedness. Fall is a time when anxieties have a tendency to increase, and our energy feels scattered. It's as if the wind creates an atmosphere of upheaval and uncertainty. So, for fall, the perfect mime exercise is to take on the wind—to feel what it is like to face the wind, to move into it, to push against it, to show strength even in the face of its force, and to be reverent.

Imagine there is a great, huge, massive wind. A wind so intense that if you were to hold an umbrella, it would turn inside out. Now, stand firmly in the wind even as it blows. Push against the wind. Try to walk in the wind, imagining both its strength and the strength you need to walk through it. If you get knocked down, get back up and keep walking. Have a destination so important in mind that no matter what, you are going to walk through this tremendous wind to get there. Really get into it with you entire body: imagine the wind in your hair and the resistance the wind has on your torso and legs as you move them forward. What is the temperature of the wind? What does the wind sound like? Can you hear the trees rustling? Is your hair whipping against your face?

Imagine the wind is your worries, your anxiety, your fears. Push into it, move through it. Show strength in the windstorm of adversity. Now imagine the wind has stopped. It is quiet and still and calm. Raise your head up and look around imagining you have arrived where you need to be.

Tree Pose

Tree Pose is a great way of working with balance, learning to sway with the winds of life, and of opening the hips, which is where we store old emotions.

Start at the top of your mat, feet hips' width apart. Feel your feet rooted down on your mat at three points: under the ridge under your big toe, the ridge under your pinky toe, and at the center of your heel. Allow your toes to wiggle, even as the rest of your feet ground down.

Keeping your right foot grounded down, begin to let your left foot slowly lift. You have many options here—you can simply kickstand your left foot; bring the bottom of your left foot to rest on your right calf; or bring it to the inside of your right thigh. Just make sure that your left foot is not placed on your knee. Keep your breath smooth and steady. You may feel yourself sway—that's great! Feel how strong you are rooted down even as you sway.

You may take your hands to your hips; lift your arms over your head, palms facing in toward each other; reach your arms out into a V shape and float them like branches to your tree; or any other formation that feels right to you. See whether you can open your hips a bit more by drawing your left knee toward the back of the room.

After several rounds of breath, lower your arms through center to your side and lower your elevated foot to the ground. Repeat on the other side.

Warrior 3

Warrior 3 improves memory and concentration so you can focus on what really matters and let go more easily of what no longer serves you. We will start this pose much as we started Tree Pose, by feeling our feet root down in those three points: under the ridge under your big toe, the ridge under your pinkie toe, and at the center of your heel.

Lift your arms overhead, palms facing in, shoulder blades drawn down to create a long neck. As you continue to root down through the right foot, begin to slowly let the left foot float off of the ground as you hinge forward at your waist. Continue leaning forward, reaching your arms and torso toward the front of the room as you extend your left leg toward the back of the room to create a straight line from your fingertips all the way back to your heel.

Keep your breath deep, slow, and even to help you balance. See whether you can even out your hips. Point your left toes straight down toward the ground.

After several breaths, take one final inhale and slowly bring your left foot back to the mat, returning to your starting position, arms at your side. Take a moment and repeat on the other side.

Legs up the Wall

This season is all about letting go and releasing, and there are few better ways to do this than Legs up the Wall.

This pose is exactly what it sounds like, so start by taking the narrow end of your yoga mat and placing it flush with a wall. If you would like to elevate your hips a little bit (purely optional based on what works best for you), bring either a folded blanket or bolster up to the edge of the wall at the bottom of your mat.

Legs up the Wall can be a bit awkward to get into, but once you're situated, it's pure comfort and relaxation. Bring yourself to sit sideways on the mat, blanket, or bolster so that the right side of your hip and thigh are right against the wall. One little movement at a time, maneuver yourself from there so that your hips stay close to the wall as you center your back on the mat and lie back. In the end, you should be in sort of an L shape, with your back on the mat and your legs—surprise, surprise—up the wall. You should exert no effort here as the wall supports the weight of your legs, doing the work of this inversion for you.

Close your eyes, let your breath come naturally, and remain in this position for as long as you would like. Enjoy!

all-seasonal movements: unwind

Admittedly, these all-season movements aren't actually movements at all. They are alternative means of generating and restoring energy on those days and in those moments when you simply don't have any energy in you.

Yoga Nidra

Yoga Nidra doesn't involve any Downward Dogs or Warrior poses. Yoga Nidra is a state of consciousness. Specifically, it is that state that exists between waking and sleeping. Yoga Nidra leaves in its wake the restoration of both mental and physical strength. When practiced over time, it illuminates where we are holding tension and helps us release the tension naturally, even when we're *not* practicing Yoga Nidra.

The objective of Yoga Nidra is to relax with awareness—gently, subtly, and consciously relaxing the body and mind. It is natural to be distracted by random thoughts during this practice. Do not try to curb them. Allow them to come and go without judgment. Tell yourself that you will not fall asleep while doing this practice. If you do fall asleep, that's okay, but the idea is to get to a place where you are in between the waking and sleeping states. With frequent practice you will be able to achieve this state.

Before beginning your practice, set an intention. This should be whatever it is your heart desires, stated in the present tense. Repeat this statement to yourself three times. It is like planting a seed in the soil of you that will continue to grow even in your waking state. You will find that during your waking state, this statement will spontaneously appear in your mind and it is always a pleasant and uplifting surprise.

Once you have finished setting your intention, in your comfortable and relaxed position either lying on a yoga mat or on your bed, allow your bones and muscles to sink deeply into the earth. Close your eyes and release yourself, let everything go. You are about to embark on a full body scan.

Take a few slow, deep, relaxed breaths. Notice the sounds in the distance and now bring your attention to the sounds in the space where you are, and then bring your attention back to your breath.

When you are ready, gently take your attention to your right foot. Do not concentrate or focus on what a foot is, touch it, or move it, just simply and gently bring your attention to your foot and acknowledge it. Gently move your attention up to your right knee, right thigh, and hip. Become aware of your whole right leg. Repeat this process for your left leg.

Next, move your attention up through your genitals, belly, and chest. Take your attention to your right shoulder and right arm, palms, and fingers, then repeat this on your left shoulder and left arm, throat, face, and, finally, the top of your head.

Take a deep breath in, repeat your intention, and observe the sensations in your body, and relax in this still state for several minutes. Now, slowly becoming aware of your body and surroundings, the sounds in the room, the sounds in the larger distance, turn to whichever side feels natural and stay lying down for a few more minutes. Rolling over to your right side makes the breath flow through your left nostril, which helps cool the body, and rolling onto your left side makes the breath flow through your right nostril, which is warming. Your body will naturally know if it needs to be cooled or warmed. Taking your time, slowly sit up, and whenever you feel comfortable, slowly and gradually open your eyes. Take note of how deeply and utterly relaxed and at peace you feel.

Energy-Pulling

You've probably heard about oil pulling, but what about energy-pulling? Through this practice, we are able to correct and piece back together our fractured energy.

To begin, identify where you are feeling fragmented, out of sorts, or off of your game. Perhaps your thoughts are spiraling, your anxiety or stress levels are high, or you are feeling distracted. All of these are symptoms that your energy has been fractured, which means you need to pull it back together and into yourself.

Begin by imagining all of your energy, floating around you. Concentrate on your breath and visualize pulling all of that energy back into your spine, gathering your energy back into your epicenter. Imagine the energy traveling up and down your spine and that you have access to this energy to pull from when needed. This can be done at any time, including when you are on the move, walking around, in your car, or laying down at the beginning or end of the day.

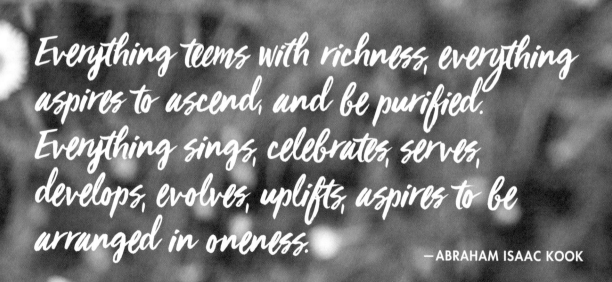

Everything teems with richness, everything aspires to ascend, and be purified. Everything sings, celebrates, serves, develops, evolves, uplifts, aspires to be arranged in oneness.

—ABRAHAM ISAAC KOOK

Part Four:

MAPPING

As we near the end of this book, we also draw closer to the real beginning of your Slow Beauty practice. I just love how endings and beginnings meld together into an infinite cycle.

As we turn our attention toward mapping, you are going to start thinking about creating a personal map for your unique journey. Here you will identify things you are already doing, aspects of this book that appeal to you, and other ideas you've heard about but haven't yet been able to incorporate into your life. This Slow Beauty practice has some external expressions, but most of the work is invisible. It happens from the inside out. This includes all of the thoughts we think and the feelings we feel. Through the practice we'll be laying out in this section, we're essentially clearing the space between ourself and our thoughts and feelings, and making sure those thoughts and feelings of ours are nontoxic, functional, natural, and beautiful.

We can think of our inner life like the interior of a home. We put so much effort into creating a safe, aesthetically pleasing, organized, healthy environment at home. Of *course* we should want the same standards for our interior home as well. Slow Beauty mapping is the act of replacing inner life estrangement with inner life engagement; with that, we design our dream home within. And guess what? You and you alone are the architect, the contractor, the subcontractors, the specialists, the interior designer, and the resident.

Some of us may only need some minor renovations within, while others will require more extensive construction. Only you will know what you need, since no one else can peek inside this interior home of yours. The approach you take to develop your map and the practice that ensues will help you see yourself, others, and life itself through a new, clearer, and sharper lens. It's as if you are looking through a pair of binoculars to see something in the distance, and you move the focusers just right and suddenly what was fuzzy and difficult to make out is clear as day. Mapping is your opportunity to chart a course to clear out the toxins, old baggage, and junk you've been hiding in the proverbial closet, and to get superfocused, purposeful, and intentional about life. And if you need to bring in the bulldozer to do some heavy lifting, well then, go for it! It's your home, after all.

I opened this chapter with one of my favorite quotes by the great mystic Kook, because when you map it out, your Slow Beauty practice engraves his ideas in your heart. Your map should do everything that he describes; it should teem with richness and inspire you to ascend and be purified. It should sing to you and celebrate you, serve and develop you, evolve and uplift you. And, most important, it should make you feel whole.

What you seek is seeking you. —RUMI

unpack your tool kit

find your guides

Through your intuition, *you* are your one and only true guide, guru, and master of your life and destiny. Any other type of guide is purely an inspirational one (which, of course, is always a good thing). In this section, we will identify those people who act as a source of light and inspiration in our life. These are the people who exemplify qualities that we would like to awaken within ourself. For example, Einstein might be a guide because he personifies a youthful spirit of wonder. Or perhaps your grandmother is because of her resilience.

You can also think of this as a process of selecting your own personal board of trustees or advisory council. Keeping these people in mind and identifying why they're important and worthy of emulation gives us a touchstone, both on a moment-by-moment basis and in those situations when we're making key decisions.

Guides are archetypes. They are akin to invisible energies that exist across cultures, and in our collective consciousness. They are a collection of our myths, experiences, histories, and beliefs. All are alive and accessible to us, regardless of our limited perspective of death. Their imprints live on.

For a bit of inspiration, here are some of my guides and their credentials. I consult with them often through their writings, teachings, poetry, music, and imagery.

Albert Einstein

Albert Einstein embodies the spirit of neoteny, from the Latin for "holding youth." Einstein had a youthful, playful spirit that was part of his genius. He lived in a state of awe and wonder. He approached, questioned, and prodded the world around him like a little child with fresh, curious eyes. Einstein was always growing young. And he was absolutely brilliant.

Rumi

The mystic poet Rumi is a deeply heralded guide because he proposes that we see with our heart. We think of the brain as the center of knowledge and believe that the more information we amass, the wiser we will be. What scientists have now discovered and are researching further is that knowledge is gathered and processed from a committee of various organs that work together to inform us, including the brain, heart, and liver. Rumi figured this out long ago.

Rachel Carson

Ecologist Rachel Carson was always interested in the whole. Her beloved book *Silent Spring* (1962), inspired a generation of environmental activists, and continues to inspire generations to think about their relationship with the natural world. Her work reminds us that we, along with all living creatures, are part of a vast interdependent ecosystem. We are responsible for one another's well-being. Each of us holds the keys to the kingdom.

Vesta

Vesta, the Roman goddess of hearth, home, and family and keeper of the sacred flame, teaches us how to care for ourself and how to keep things warm and cozy at home. She is the one who makes sure the fire is always burning.

David Bowie

Bowie overflowed with rich creativity. His approach to death was no different than how he approached anything else in life. Bowie's final album was an expression of his feelings and thoughts about his impending death, and ultimately about the true beauty of life. He lived at the highest rung of Diotima's ladder, the rung of the form of beauty.

Okay, so I guess when it comes to my guides, "I see dead people." But even though they're deceased, these incredible people have so much to share with us that we keep them alive within us. Psychologist Abraham Maslow advises us to "study healthy people." He says, "The study of such healthy people can teach us much about our own mistakes, our shortcomings, the proper directions in which to grow. Every age has had its model, its ideal. All these have been given up by culture: the saint, the hero, the knight, the mystic." Let's go against the grain and not give up on these ideals. Let's identify them and learn from them.

Take stock of who you are "studying." We do this unconsciously every day. We "study" celebrities, friends, and family members. Studying is another form of ingesting, and digesting. Make sure you are studying healthy people so you benefit from their elevated knowledge and way of becoming. There is a reason we become attracted to certain guides and not others. The attraction has to do with an aspect of the psychological patterning they embody, what Jung refers to as an "archaic remnant" that represents itself to us as an "archetypal motif," an image that contains patterns residing in the universal collective unconscious waiting to be actualized by the person undergoing the individuation process. Integration of the characteristics of guides who inspire you will awaken more available resources within and lead you to strengthening your most important and relevant guide—*you!*

Think about who resonates deeply with you, be it an author, politician, poet, performer, friend, or family member. It could be anyone whose qualities, values, and characteristics move and profoundly affect you. Write their names down here and underneath their name write down their credentials and the reason why they belong on your personal advisory council. Plot this information into your map.

your consort ganesh: a coloring meditation

Coloring is always a wonderful way to slow down and get in touch with our creativity. All the better if we're channeling our focus into inspirational symbols like Ganesh, known as the remover of obstacles!

How many obstacles did Oprah have to overcome? Gandhi? Martin Luther King Jr.? How many obstacles have *you* overcome? And how many more will there be? But even more than the number of obstacles we encounter in life, is how we face and displace them. Some obstacles need to be dissolved, others knocked down, some climbed over, and, still others, pushed through. The point is that, whatever it takes, we must prevail. What if Oprah, Gandhi, and Martin Luther King Jr. had given up? Be tenacious. When an obstacle shows up—and they *will*, over and over again—understand them as the force that refines us. Acknowledge them, face them, and call upon Ganesh to assist you in transforming the obstacles

into your light. Think of it as a video game: An obstacle appears, you conquer it, the obstacle dissolves, and a light that now belongs to you appears in its place. The more obstacles you confront and conquer, the more light you collect.

Ganesh is like the guardian angel of obstacles, the large, strong elephant that obliterates obstacles so you can move onward. Do this coloring meditation to integrate the concept of Ganesh into your psyche. The next time an obstacle arises, recall and repeat this simple meditative mantra: *Ganesh, Ganesh, Ganesh.* It's a bit like "there's no place like home" or "bibbidi, bobbidi, boo." If Ganesh isn't your thing, create your own mantra to utilize the next time an obstacle appears in your life. Be sure to write it here on this page and in your map so you can refer to it later. This is your magic song to be sung when the obstacles appear. And through the singing you, not the obstacle, will prevail.

animal medicine

In Native American culture, it is believed that animals represent certain qualities. For example, ant medicine represents endurance, patience, and persistence; lizards symbolize transformation and regrowth. When an animal appears to us on a regular or synchronistic basis, it is revealing its medicine to us. In this section, we will take the time to slow down and take stock of the animal

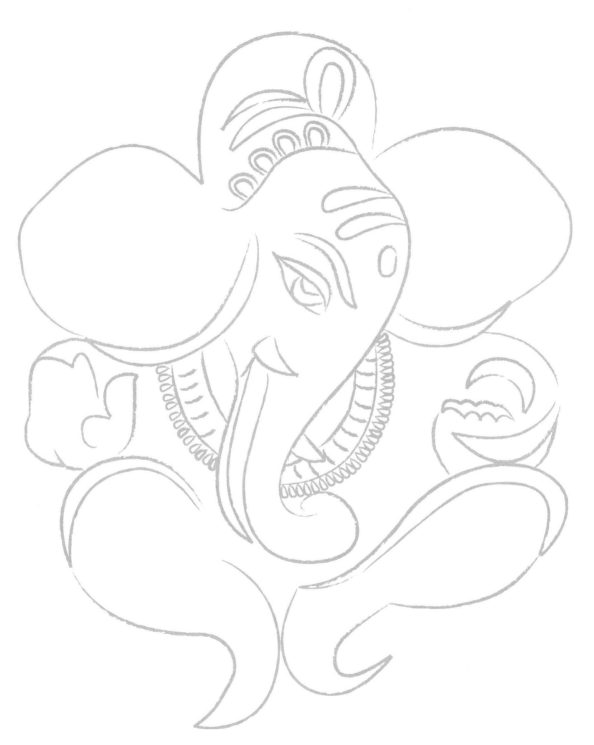

medicine that is appearing in own life, gain an understanding of what that medicine symbolizes, and how it might be applied to our life.

Pay attention to what shows up in your waking life. When Torti the tortoise came to live with us for two weeks, his presence inspired an entire philosophy of beauty that I now share with you. When an animal or insect crosses your path, pay attention and do a little research on what they symbolize in both Native American and other cultures. Paying attention to details like this helps us to be more present in our life. The medicine specific animals contain may inspire you or reveal the answer to a question you've been asking.

Mostly, the presence of an insect or an animal—no matter how brief—can be quite magical if we allow it to be. Acknowledging nature, rather than just taking it for granted as we move about our daily activities, helps us connect with and honor the beauty and wonder of the world around us. The purpose of honoring the insects and animals is to hone our own perception and, ultimately, to strengthen our intuition for clarity and self-knowledge. Nature is so much a part of our daily life, yet we have blinders on that keep us zoned in on our narrow sense of self (and in our "smart" devices). Once we catch a glimpse of the beauty of nature, and then another, and then get to the point where we seek it out, we will remove those blinders and expand our vision of ourself. We will experience moments of wonder. Indeed, making this connection with nature is a vital part of growing young.

The following are a few examples of animals and insects and what they represent. Should an animal or insect appear in your life that isn't included here, a quick search from one of the following resources will illuminate their meaning: *Animal Speak* by Ted Andrews is an amazing reference book to keep on hand. Online, I like whats-your-sign.com, spirit-animals.com, and spiritanimal.info. I encourage you to delve deeper into any animal that shows up often in your life or with which you have always felt a special connection. If there is a particular animal with which you feel connected, consider surrounding yourself with visual images of this animal and keep it close. If you have always felt a kinship with a certain animal or insect, it is definitely worth a deeper exploration to learn how their specific power or energy is meant to support you and nourish you. The following are examples of animals and their significance to get you started. Be sure to include images of creatures from the natural kingdom that "speak" to you on your map.

BUTTERFLY

Joy, joy, and more joy! The medicine of the butterfly is all about elevation and the lightness of being. It is about being in flight with self-expression and creativity. It shows us that work, commitment, and dedication will transform into something artful and elegant.

CATERPILLAR

These insects represent potential of the purest kind. They remind us that the work we are doing—the preparing, the thinking, the information—are all working together to soon be transformed into something completely new and colorful. We only need to have patience to make it through this gestation period before the rebirth. Be patient. Be tenacious. That is what the caterpillar is communicating.

DEER

Deer remind us of grace. Their swiftness and humility demonstrate how to even out our temperament should it be excessive in one direction. If a deer appears to you, it's a reminder to return to love and peace, and to perform random acts of loving kindness and compassion.

EAGLE

When you spot an eagle, chances are it is high up in the sky. Eagle medicine is about higher thought vibrations and freedom from the mental blocks and prisons in which we trap ourself. Have you heard the expression "eagle eye"? Eagles have precise eyesight and thus remind us to stay laser-focused on what we need to accomplish. No distractions allowed!

FIREFLY

The firefly is a magical creature that illuminates our path in the darkness. Their light bounces and dances around. When we come across fireflies, it is medicine for new ideas, inspiration, and creativity—kind of like the flickering lightbulb of that new formula you've just discovered!

HUMMINGBIRD

These tiny birds teach us how to tap into the infinite wellspring of joy. When a hummingbird shows up in your life, it is a reminder that joy resides within. Perhaps you have lost sight of this. If so, the hummingbird's high vibration wing movement in the pattern of a figure eight is here to remind you to reorient yourself toward joy.

LIZARD

Highly sensitive and perceptive, the lizard is closely related to intuition and appears to remind you to let your intuition guide you. There are messages waiting in your dreamtime that you should pay close attention to. Lizard also symbolizes our ability to regenerate that which has been lost. Because of its tail-removing ability, it is a master at diversion when in dangerous situations. Use that technique to aid you when you are feeling threatened.

PRAYING MANTIS

In almost all cultures, this creature is a symbol of stillness. When a mantis appears to you, it is time to retreat to a quiet place and to get back in touch with your intuition. If you have been overactive and feel unbalanced, the medicine of the praying mantis is telling you to slow down and find moments of peace and calm.

RAVEN

The magical raven has something to tell us about the deep mysteries of self. They are highly intelligent birds and, according to Carl Jung, their medicine represents the shadow aspects of ourself—those deep, mysterious aspects we need to draw near to experience a sense of wholeness. When a raven appears, take it as a sign that an aspect of yourself that you have kept in the dark is about to be revealed.

ROOSTER

Roosters appear as a wake-up call. Where are you asleep in your life? Time to wake up and get some work done. They are full of activity, ever watchful, and their eccentricity reminds us that it is okay to be playful and colorful.

SNAKE

Snakes show us how to set clear intentions for impending changes. As snakes shed their skin, so do we. We have the ability to reinvent ourself, to begin anew. A snake gives us permission to shed that which no longer serves us. It helps us tap into our energy trove, our life force, to process this transformation. When a snake shows up, it is a powerful message that a big, transformative change is possible in your life.

SPARROW

The sparrow represents connection with the spiritual realm. Sparrows travel in groups, so they are also representative of strength in numbers. If a sparrow shows up, ask yourself if you need to spend more time in the warmth of good friends, or perhaps to reconnect with your spirit. Sparrow is also a symbol of inclusion. In what ways have you excluded parts of yourself?

WOODPECKER

The most specific message a woodpecker has is about discrimination. Are you being discerning in the decisions you are currently making in your life or are you just jumping right in without taking the time for reflection? The woodpecker is a reminder to use your head and figure out solutions that feel right before moving forward.

ABRACADABRA:
I Create What I Speak

Words have meaning. They have an origin and a history. It is important that we choose our words wisely. We should research them to better understand and imbue them with more meaning. Your vocabulary is yours and yours alone. Perhaps you have adopted some words and phrases that don't quite fit you or the person you want to be. Perhaps you inherited them from your upbringing; they've been passed down from generation to generation and are therefore familiar to you, but not generative, expansive, or transformative. Identify the words and phrases you use that don't actually belong to you and remove them from your vocabulary. You can do this by sitting with a familiar phrase and noticing how it makes you feel. If it feels heavy, weighted, or stifling, then transform it. You create what you speak, so we have a big responsibility to become conscious of what statements we are making out in the world.

Think about phrases you use on a regular basis. Write them here. Don't judge them—get them all out in broad daylight and then transform the ones that feel heavy into a phrase that is more generative, useful, and supportive.

_____

_____

_____

_____

_____

_____

_____

_____

_____

_____

There is a form of communication called Nonviolent Communication (NVC), developed by Dr. Marshall B. Rosenberg. It is a form of communication that uses language in a specific way to communicate compassionately. The main guiding principles of NVC are observations, feelings, empathy, and self-empathy. NVC has identified certain feelings we experience when our needs are being met, and other feelings we experience when they are not. Our human needs are universal, and it is our birthright to be in a safe environment where we are able to meet our needs. One way to accomplish this is to take responsibility for how we communicate with our self and others. If we have a tendency to communicate in a violent manner due to cultural conditioning or any other factors, we now have the opportunity to change our language so that it is more compatible with our needs and the needs of others in our life.

NVC teaches us:

(1) To observe, not judge. Describe a situation without labeling it. Instead of "He is a yelling tyrant who never listens to what I'm saying," say, "He is yelling right now and isn't in a place to listen to what I have to say."

(2) Identify your feelings. Instead of "I feel manipulated into doing what he wants me to do," try "I feel frustrated. I don't think I'm going to have an opportunity to express what I'd like to share."

(3) State your needs. Instead of "I feel frustrated because you aren't listening to me," say, "I feel frustrated because I need your support."

(4) Ask for what you want clearly. State, "Would you be willing to hear what I have to say without interrupting me?" instead of "Would you make sure not to raise your voice to me again?"

(5) Have empathy for others. NVC points out that often we are not in a place to offer the right words, but we can be empathic toward the person with whom we would like to communicate in a peaceful manner. According to the method of NVC, empathy is something that can be offered silently and wordlessly.

(6) Have empathy for yourself. Self-empathy is when we listen deeply to our personal needs and feelings. This will help us to determine what our next step will be.

With all of this in mind, I would like you to select and brainstorm words that really resonate, connect with, and inspire you. Following are a few words to get your collection going. Add to them as you find words that resonate with you. Then, *use* those words. Make a concerted effort to slip them into conversation and writing. Study them. Proclaim them. Love them. Enjoy and enjoin them. When you're in the mood to hunt down some new words, the online Etymology Dictionary (ety-monline.com) is a good resource, as is the Visual Thesaurus (visualthesaurus.com). These sites will tell you everything you need to know about the birth and origin of the words in your collection. It's nice to know someone from the day they are born! Once you've found your words and put them to use, watch how they come alive in your life.

Here is an example to get you started:

JOYOUS

Joyous was born in France in the 1300s. It is an adjective that comes from the French word *joios*, which means "cheerful, happy." Synonyms of *joyous* include amused, delighted, and happy. *Joyous*

is a word I hold often, and a state of being I one day realized perfectly described what I needed, how I wanted to feel in the world every day. The joy isn't always large and I don't always wear it on my face, but it is a constant. And when I feel a bit down, I remember the joy I've found within and I kindle the flame a bit to turn it up.

That's it! Make a list of your words, jot down their origin, and some thoughts and feelings you have about the particular word. Use the words when you are out in the world. Use them when you speak to yourself.

Here are some other words that may resonate with you and that you may want to incorporate into your collection:

affectionate	grateful	love
engaged	hopeful	magnanimous
evolution	inspired	peaceful
excited	liberation	refreshed
exhilarated	light	visceral

What if each word we spoke was a blessing we put into the world? Think about the words you are going to speak before you say them. Make your language generative, expansive, and supportive to both yourself and to others. Speak poetically about yourself and others. When you speak, you are concretizing ideas. You are giving them a form that lives in the world, in someone's ear, settles in their mind, and that may one day flow from their lips. Choose your words wisely.

METAPHORS AS MUSE

A metaphor is a representation or symbol of something else, such as "all the world's a stage," (Shakespeare) or "chaos is a friend of mine" (Bob Dylan). I believe that much of the language we use, the words we exchange with others, and the words that compose the thoughts we think, could become a barrier to our natural process when those words we say and think don't serve our higher purpose. We get entangled in these words and they become our belief system. They become "words to live by." Metaphors help shake us up a bit. They move us outside of our cemented perspectives and help us see things in new ways—in ways that help us be more creative. And when we are more creative, we are better able to problem-solve and to develop skills that are helpful to us and to the world around us.

Metaphors transport us to a deeper place, a more profound state of being, and thinking, feeling, and living. We've lost the art of the metaphor, and with it the art of conversation and the art of being still long enough to go a little deeper. I use metaphors in my life as a tool to help reconnect me with a secret, poetic interior language that binds me to life in a deeper, more meaningful way. Metaphors are a vehicle for reaching those deeper states of being. In fact, this Slow Beauty map is a metaphor that connects us more deeply with our needs.

See how you can incorporate metaphors into your own language and notice the effect it has on you and your connection with the world around you.

create your own soundtrack

Listening to music heals us mentally, emotionally, and even physically by calming our nervous system. Without even thinking about it, our body starts to release and move to the rhythm of the music. It's kind of amazing when you think about it.

Following are some music recommendations to move you. They are categorized by season based on the mood the genre evokes. I realize that musical tastes are extremely personal, so I encourage you to develop your very own soundtrack for each season. You can use the list of albums that have moved me over the years as a starting point if you're looking for inspiration.

As you create your soundtrack, select music that moves you and takes you on a profound journey. Music is unparalleled in its power to lift us up and set us down, to bring us to a state of ecstasy, to warm us, and to soothe. Music has the ability to reach deep inside us, touch us, and hold us. The perfect combination of sounds, cadence, rhythm, and lyrics elevate our senses, they make us think, and they arrest our thoughts. Songs mark moments in our life. They remind us of where we've been, and encourage us to go where we need to be. They conjure up memories, and relationships both distant and present. When we connect with a song or an album, it becomes like a trusted and true friend who we can call upon in our times of need. Music makes the world go round.

Of course, nowadays it's easiest to download music onto our devices, but I do recommend investing in a record player and some vinyl to reap the benefits of analog sound, which is much more appealing and healing for the ear. We are bombarded with digital sound and it is nice to give our ears a rest from this type of sound whenever possible. Think of it as a digital detox for your ear canal!

WINTER: GO DEEP

Winter is a time of year when we can become quiet and slightly withdrawn. It is a season in which we are offered the time to reflect and envision in preparation for the burst of excitement that comes with spring. That makes winter the perfect season to spend some one-on-one time with various types of instruments. I find this variety is exactly what I need to keep things stimulating when my feelings and moods may become a bit lackluster during the winter months.

For the winter playlist I've selected a diverse repertoire that includes a harp, a cello, a piano, and a banjo (played by Steve Martin, no less!).

Inspire: Evelyn Huber
Songs from the Arc of Life: Yo-Yo Ma
Countdown: Joey Alexander
Rare Bird Alert: Steve Martin and the Steep
    Canyon Rangers

SPRING: JAZZ

In spring everything is all aflutter, blooming, and bursting. It is the season of spontaneity, excitement, and buzz. Jazz is the perfect genre to elicit feelings of springtime, because of its fluid, improvisational essence. There are so many incredible jazz albums that it's difficult to choose just a few. Nonetheless, here is a short list to get you started.

A Love Supreme: John Coltrane
Kind of Blue: Miles Davis
Ellington at Newport: Duke Ellington
A Boy Named Charlie Brown: Vince Guaraldi Trio
Mo' Better Blues Soundtrack: Branford Marsalis
    and Terence Blanchard
Straight No Chaser: Thelonious Monk
Saxophone Colossus: Sonny Rollins

SUMMER: SOUL

Summer is warm, languid, and passionate. Summer is soulful. What better time of the year to delve into the greatest soul musicians of all time, to connect with the soul of our summer season?

Lady Soul: Aretha Franklin
What's Going On: Marvin Gaye
Otis Blue: Otis Redding
Nina Simone Sings the Blues: Nina Simone
Songs in the Key of Life: Stevie Wonder
Inner Visions: Stevie Wonder

FALL: SINGER-SONGWRITER

Fall is a very poetic time of year as the changing leaves fall from the trees and into colorful piles on the ground beneath them. There is something so lyrical about fall, so what better music to explore than those singer-songwriters whose lyrics reach into us and transform us?

Rubber Soul: The Beatles
Leonard Cohen: Leonard Cohen
Blood on the Tracks: Bob Dylan
Tumbleweed Connection: Elton John
Tapestry: Carole King
Semper Femina: Laura Marling
Blue: Joni Mitchell
Harold and Maude Soundtrack: Various artists

shapeshifting

This playful exercise will allow you to see yourself in new and more expansive ways. You will find that these prompts aren't in any particular order, and that is on purpose. It is meant to be illogical and nonsensical, to shake up the linear, practical, rigid part of the brain that often keeps us stuck in our comfort zone. This is an improvisational exercise meant to be done quickly. Don't overthink it; just fill in the blanks with whatever comes to mind. The more absurd the better. When you are done filling in the prompts, try to draw or collage this portrait of yourself. When you see it all come together, what is it that you really see?

If I were a plant, I would be a _____, and if I had to choose a material out of which to build my home it would be _____. The shape of my home would be _____. If I were a composite animal, my eyes would be that of a _____, my ears that of a _____, my torso that of a _____, my legs that of a _____, my feet that of a _____, and my hands that of a _____. If I were a sound, I would sound like a _____ and you would hear me in the _____. When I move, I move like _____. My dance of choice is the _____. If I were to paint myself a color from head to toe, it would be _____. If I were a weather condition, I would be _____. I am the season _____. If I were a feeling, I would be _____. When the wind blows it _____ me, and when it rains I _____. Ice _____ when I touch it. When I come across a meadow I _____. There is a gift waiting for me in the meadow. I unwrap it and find _____, and then I _____. Someone is walking toward me and they are _____ and I _____. I like to _____.

I am a _____ tree. If I were a language I would be _____. If I had my own country it would be called _____. If I were a symbol I would be the symbol _____.

The next time you find yourself in a boring situation, try to recall some of these answers. Imagine that you *are* the plant, or touching ice. Allow your imagination to run free, bringing more playfulness, open-mindedness, flexibility, and humor into your life.

remember a slower time

If you find that slowing down is difficult for you to do, don't worry. You're not alone. It takes some practice in this modern world we live in. More and more, it's easy to forget that we're not doing something wrong if we *do* stop. There's always e-mail to answer, errands to run, Netflix to watch. We are surrounded by communication, information, and entertainment at all times. It can feel like a barrage. Even if our body can slow down, getting our brain to follow suit is an entirely different matter.

To avoid getting swept up in this fixation on busy-ness, it's important to remind ourself that this is not how we were made. It's not how we were meant to live. Think about how the world worked at pretty much any point in history up until a little over one hundred years ago.

Since there were no alarm clocks, you would wake up with the sun and perhaps some animals as your cue. Breakfast—and all of your nourishment, for that matter—would consist of whatever was seasonal and available. "Work" likely blended in with life in general, involved tasks around the home and your land. It's likely that at least some of this work was outdoors, so that you could soak up sunshine and fresh air as you completed your tasks. You moved from one undertaking to another, one at a time. There was no multitasking or incessant stops and starts due to rings and vibrations and pings coming from the phone in your pocket. In fact, I'm willing to bet that work was actually quite meditative because it was uninterrupted.

Your day would likely finish with the setting sun. You would perhaps spend some time with your loved ones by the light of a fire and some candles. Your entertainment for the evening was one another. Before long, after a day of working and without artificial light, it was time for a fitful, uninterrupted night's rest until morning light came around again.

Remember who you are and how you were made. Slowing down is your birthright. You were never built to be on hyperdrive.

YOU ARE HERE

You've identified your guides and your language; you've packed your medicine and you have the idea of Ganesh at the forefront of your mind to help you crush obstacles along your way. You know how to shapeshift when necessary. You have your objective—to retrieve your light, your essence. Yes, many of the rituals and recipes in this book will help your skin glow, but, really, it is the light you are igniting to illuminate the bridge between your conscious and unconscious self that will radiate the most intensely. As Joseph Campbell points out in *Hero with a Thousand Faces*, it is there in the unconscious where the meaning resides. So you will need to travel there to find the meaning and bring it back.

This entire book has been leading up to this mapping exercise. Each page represents a season and includes an illustration of a tree that you may color and add onto with your own design. These trees are a metaphor for how we connect with our own natural seasons and how we ground down, expand, grow, and let go. You will "decorate" your tree for each season by plotting out the recipes, rituals, strategies, and tactics that will guide you through the season at hand. This Slow Beauty Mapping exercise will help you become more self-aware and self-accepting as you move through the various cycles of life. Use the tree to plot out the recipes, rituals, and exercises you would like to integrate into your life each season. You can pull from what you like in this book as well as plotting out things you are already doing in your life and ideas you've read or heard about but haven't yet had the opportunity to incorporate.

Stay positive as you make lists of things you would like to incorporate into your life, and be sure to choose things that are right for you, that speak to you, inspire you, and resonate with you. You are the visionary of your life. Make your strategic plan come to life on these pages, and then simply follow what you've mapped out.

Beauty is the gateway to having an expansive experience of life. When you see beauty both within and without, you can be assured that you are in a very good place. This process will get you to that place where you feel and see beauty everywhere. It is a way of retrieving those things that have been buried over a long period of time, whether it be because of neglect, fragmentation, numbness, a lack of discernment, or fear. The entire concept of Slow Beauty is a type of initiation to reclaim and reset what is rightfully yours—your intuition, your beauty, your rhythm, your best self.

becoming a cartographer

To plot out your map, you will need some tools and resources to assist you in surveying, analyzing, and making a connection to the lay of the land. I've included several exercises that will serve as tools to support you as you plot out your practice by season, each of which is represented by a tree. Trees have roots and serve as a great reminder of the truth "As above so below, and so below as above." Treat, heal, and purify the deep roots below, and the health of the roots will be apparent above. You will identify the knowledge you will need to access each season to help you attain the optimum level of health and beauty, and plot it on the tree and in the surrounding landscape.

The tree represents a present state of mind. Because we are often plagued by issues from our past and concerns and worries about the future, there is space around the tree to identify those challenges as well so you can face them and transform them. Your Slow Beauty map is a representation of your personal beauty standard, where you are, and where you want to be. You will create an embodied map—a map based on the qualities you would like to integrate and express, the feelings and thoughts you choose to think and feel, and the rituals and recipes you choose to integrate into your life. Mapping all of this out will philosophically and purposefully root you in your Slow Beauty practice.

getting started

STEP 1:
PHILOSOPHY

The Slow Beauty philosophy is multifaceted. To begin, zero in on the top three ideas that stand out for you from the Philosophy section (see page 15). These will serve as your three Imperatives as you plot out your map. Write them down in the illustration of each of the trees to remind you what your Slow Beauty goals are for each season. It's likely these imperatives will vary a bit from season to season, and that's good. Seasons change, and so should your imperatives. To help you hone in on the three Imperatives each season, ask yourself this question: "What do I need?" Use the *Growing Young* needs (see page 25) as a guideline to hone in on your necessities for each season.

STEP 2:
SELECT YOUR RECIPES
AND RITUALS

Identify the self-care recipes and rituals that you would like to try. These can include those found in this book, they may be rituals and recipes that you are already incorporating into your life, or those that you have been wanting to try out. These are the strategies you will be enacting to support the actualization of your three Imperatives.

STEP 3:
CREATE YOUR ACTION PLAN

Using that list of recipes and rituals you selected, apply those that you will be using in a specific season to their corresponding tree. This is the tactical portion of Slow Beauty mapping—your specific action plan for each season.

STEP 4:
TOOL KIT

You will need some tools for your journey, so I've provided a tool kit on the following pages for you to unpack prior to mapping. You may find that some of these approaches and exercises illuminate your mapping process and make your journey more fulfilling. Identify the tools that speak to you and include them in your mapping.

STEP 5:
KEEP ON MAPPING!

As you begin to put your Slow Beauty practice into action using the maps you have created for each season, use the seasonal pages to write down your thoughts, ideas, tools, rituals, recipes, and anything else that comes to mind. Build upon the recipes and rituals you are utilizing. Make them your own, and take time to reflect on the process of your practice. To help you chart, connect with, understand, and measure your progress, refer back to Abraham Maslow's signs of self-actualization (page 18). These will serve as signposts that the work you're doing is actually working. Also, be sure to document your thoughts and feelings as they arise. What are you thinking and feeling throughout this process? What's working for you? What isn't? Where are obstacles showing up? What feels easy and natural? What feels challenging and uncomfortable? Let it all happen—and acknowledge it all as it happens. Reflect on it and reflect on it some more. Fine tune. Refine.

AMELIA EARHART: MAPPING HER OWN COURSE

I've always been intrigued by Amelia Earhart, a woman of great courage who pursued her dreams by taking flight. In particular, I have always been fascinated by the mystery that surrounds her last voyage, from which she never returned. Until recently, this mystery remained unsolved. It was believed that Earhart had died in a plane crash somewhere over the Pacific Ocean. However, after years of investigation, the International Group for Historic Aircraft Recovery recently revealed a new theory that Earhart actually died as a heroic castaway on the island Nikumaroro, Kiribati, where she safely landed her plane.

Amelia Earhart serves as an icon for charting her own course, pursuing dreams, taking flight, bravery, tenacity, and the unconventional. It is for all of these reasons that she has always intrigued me. In her profession as a pilot, Earhart followed maps to get from one place to another. Moreover, as the first female to fly solo across the Atlantic, she mapped out her own unique place in the world. Her story is rich with symbolism, as is each of ours.

Unfortunately, also like Earhart, sometimes we all go missing. In what ways have you gone missing in your life? And in what ways will you identify and reclaim those missing pieces of yourself and bring them home?

In spite of all of the progress we have made, women, especially, have the tendency to go missing. We find ourself apologizing for our needs, for who we are, pleading for time for ourself, for time to pursue our dreams, for justice. We need to find a way to strike a balance. To harness equilibrium.

All of the needs identified by Ashley Montagu have so much resonance. These needs, our needs, our birthright, are the touchstones necessary to make our way back so that we don't die a castaway on some deserted island within. We go missing when we don't have a clear vision of what we need. We make compromises when we lack clarity. I know I've been lost along the way. I've deferred often to the pressures and demands of this systemic culture, to my parents' expectations, to the circumstances of my life, to poor decisions I've made. I've compromised too much. I haven't felt confident enough to express my needs—sometimes I haven't even known I had needs!

We women go missing when our most natural self goes missing, and is grown over with the weeds of the unbalanced, patriarchal culture in which we are planted. And then when we have a *satori* moment, when we realize "Hey, where am I?" and it dawns on us that we have misplaced our self somewhere. It is then that we turn into seekers, and can seek our true self with a tenacity, resolve, and strength of purpose like no other. Once you are in true partnership with yourself, there is no need to return ever again because you are already there.

winter

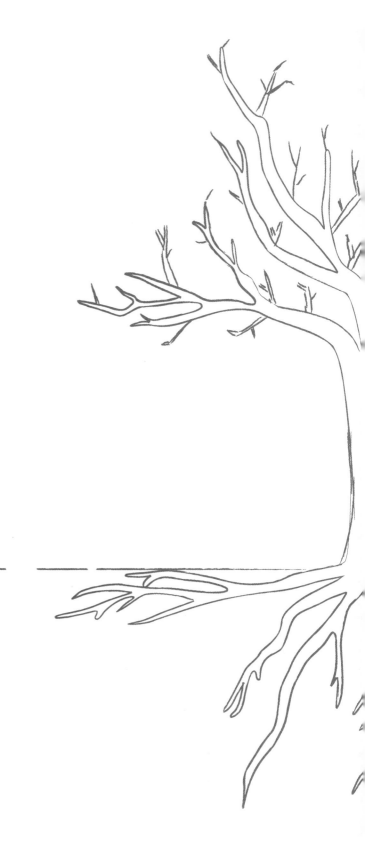

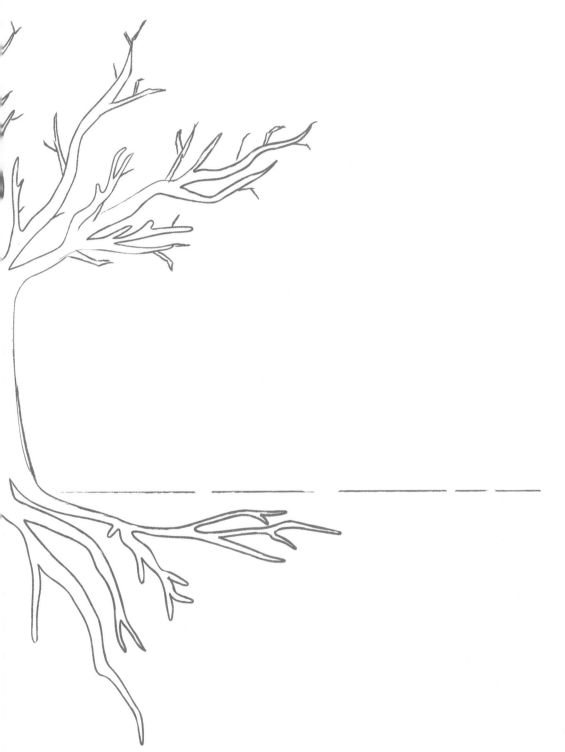

spring

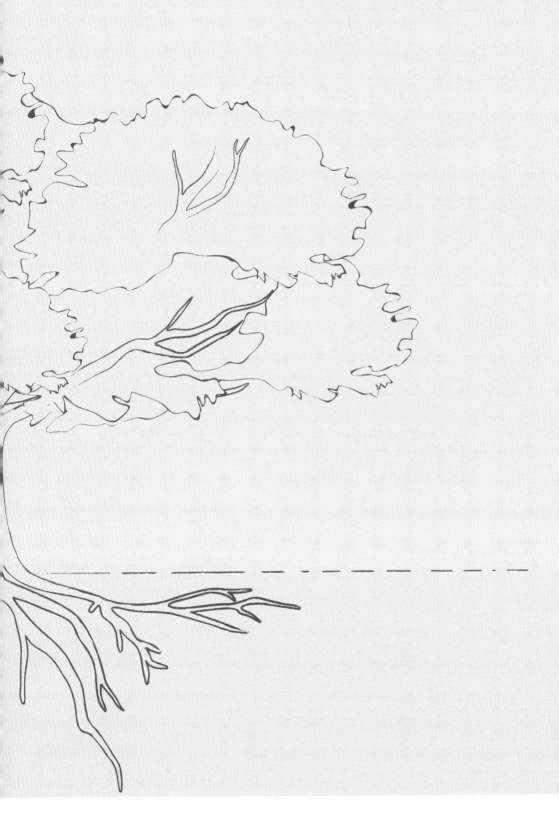

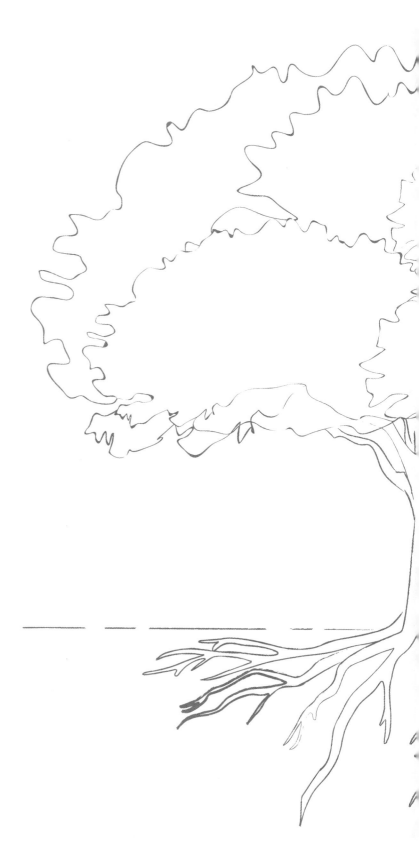

summer

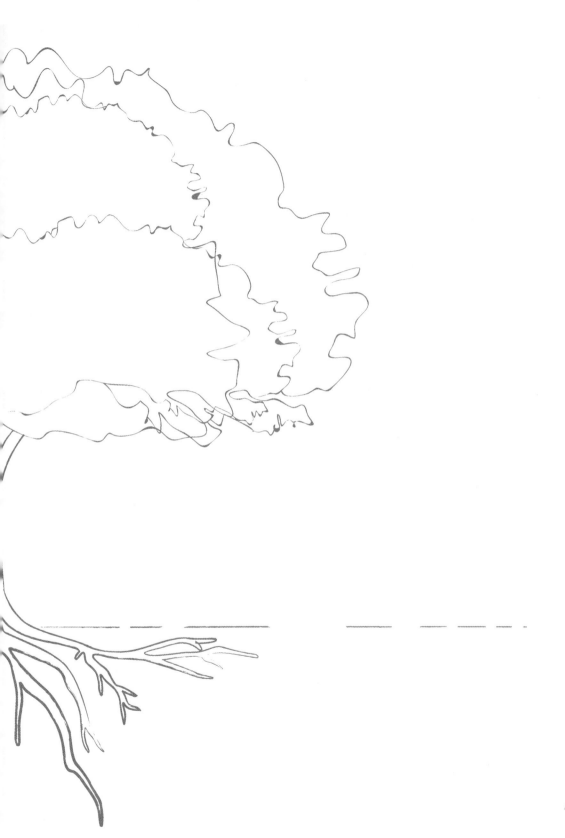

fall

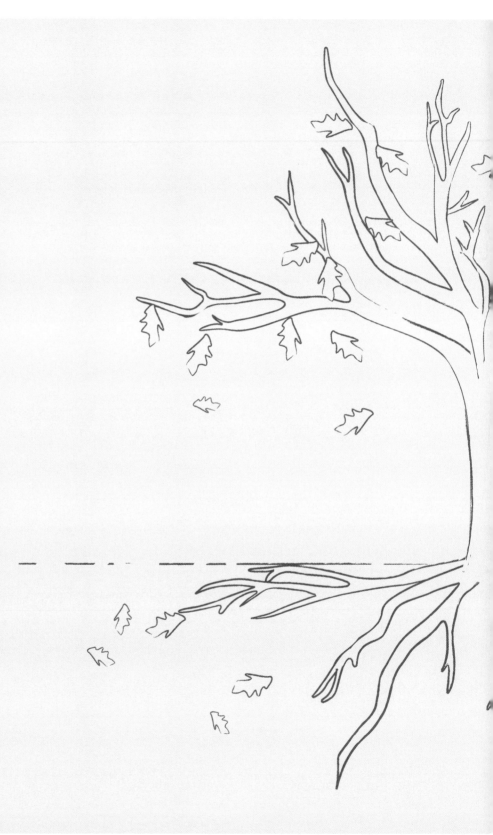

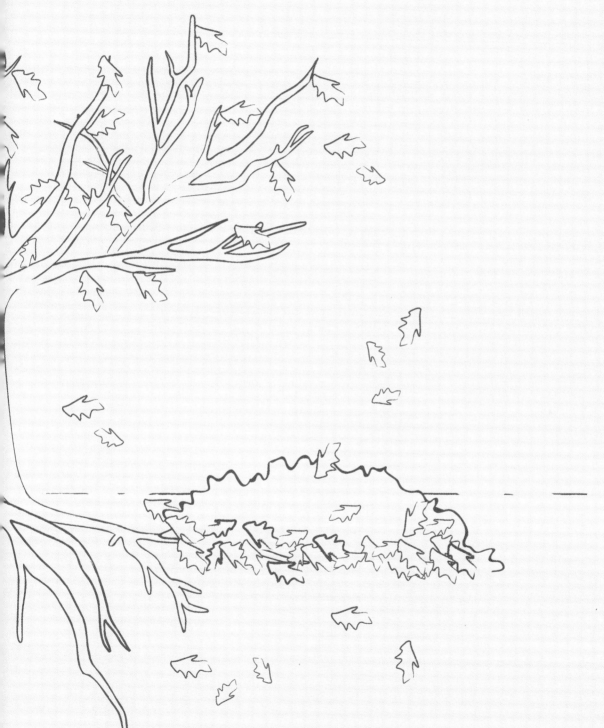

RESOURCES

The Next Enlightenment by Walter Truett Anderson; St. Martin's Press, 2003.

Animal Speak: The Spiritual and Magical Power of Creatures Great and Small by Ted Andrews; Llewellyn Publications, 2002.

Silent Spring by Rachel Carson; Houghton Mifflin Harcourt, 2002.

The Chalice and the Blade: Our History, Our Future by Riane Eisler; HarperCollins, 1988.

Women Who Run with the Wolves: Myths and Stories of the Wild Woman Archetype by Clarissa Pinkola Estés; Ballantine Books, 1992.

The Art of Loving by Erich Fromm; Bloomsbury Academic, 2000.

Last Child in the Woods: Saving Our Children from Nature-Deficit Disorder by Richard Louv; Algonquin Books, 2008.

Growing Young, 2nd Edition by Ashley Montagu; Praeger, 1988.

Anam Cara: A Book of Celtic Wisdom by John O'Donohue; Harper Perennial, 1988.

Earthing: The Most Important Health Discovery Ever by Clinton Ober; Basic Health Publications, 2014.

Symposium by Plato; Hackett Publishing Company, 1989.

From Science to God: A Physicist's Journey into the Mystery of Consciousness by Peter Russell; New World Library, 2003.

Sustainism Is the New Modernism: A Cultural Manifesto for the Sustainist Era by Michiel Schwarz and Joost Elffers; Distributed Art Publishers, 2010.

INDEX

A

action plan, creating, 206

afternoon rituals, 64–65

aging, 23–24, 91
growing young needs, 23–31, 91, 205, 211

ahbyanga, 63

alkaline water, 141, 142

almond butter pomelo winter smoothie, 130

almond milk, all-season endurance smoothie, 138

aloe vera
aloe i love you summer water, 142
beneficial properties of, 142

alternative therapies, 17–18

Anderson, Walter Truett, 19

Andrews, Ted, 193

animal medicine, 191–195

Animal Speak (Andrews), 193

apples
beneficial properties of, 133
good fortune spring smoothie, 133
tastes like apple pie fall compote, 126

apps, to connect with volunteer opportunities, 85

arm movements, in belly dancing, 175

The Artist's Way (Cameron), 177

The Art of Loving (Fromm), 35

asceticism, 94

autonomy, 19

avocado oil
beneficial properties of, 150
grapefruit avocado winter oil, 157
lavender, matcha, and avocado oil spring exfoliating powder, 150

Ayurvedic tradition, seasonal attributes and, 101–103

B

ballet positions, 176

banana, all-season endurance smoothie, 138

basil
all-season glorious greens, 129
basil, maca, and sunflower summer exfoliating powder, 153
basil cucumber summer mist, 163
beneficial properties of, 109, 126, 129
goodness in a glass summer juice, 126
pure poetry spring tea, 109

basil essential oil, basil cucumber summer mist, 163. *See also* holy basil essential oil

bathing, nature, 71–72

beauty
love as form of, 49–51
spiritualization of, 51–52
See also Slow Beauty

belly dancing, 174–175

bhramari spring breath, 171–172

bibliotherapy, 82–84
reading sets for self-actualization, 83–84

black pepper
beneficial properties of, 112, 145
classic turmeric fall tea, 112
turmeric orange fall water, 145

blood red orange
beneficial properties of, 145
turmeric orange fall water, 145

body image, 12

body oil recipes, 156–158

book club, 76

Bowie, David, 190

bowls. *See* smoothies and bowls

breathwork, 169, 170–173
breath of joy, 178
tonglen fall breath, 173

C

Cameron, Julia, 177

Campbell, Joseph, 204

Carson, Rachel, 190

caterpillar spirit animal, 194

central nervous system, consciousness and, 98

chamomile
almond butter pomelo winter smoothie, 130
beneficial properties of, 108
proper digestion winter tea, 108

chamomile essential oil
beneficial properties of, 157, 161
grapefruit avocado winter oil, 157
grapefruit chamomile winter mist, 161

change, Slow Beauty and, 39–40

chard
beneficial properties of, 117
go green spring soup, 117

Last Child in the Woods (Louv), 71

Child's Pose, 178, 180

Chinese medicine, seasonal attributes and, 101–103

"Cinderella," 33–34

classes and services, Slow Beauty practice and, 77

Cobra Pose, 180

coconut milk
beneficial properties of, 112
classic turmeric fall tea, 112

coconut sugar, in sugar scrubs, 149–154

coloring meditation, 191, 192

grapeseed oil
  beneficial properties of, 120, 149
  grapefruit, ginger, and grapeseed oil
    paste winter scrub, 149
  optimistic squash fall soup, 120

gratitude journal, 66

greens, all-season glorious greens juice,
  129. *See also* spinach

group gatherings, 11, 13, 25, 75–77

Growing Young (Montagu), 23

growing young needs, 23–31, 91, 205,
  211

guides, mapping, 189–191

H

health, beauty and, 38

health advocacy, volunteer opportunities
  for, 85

Heart Belly breathing meditation, 66

heat-generating winter breath, 171

Hero Pose, 178, 180

Hero with a Thousand Faces (Campbell), 204

hibiscus
  beneficial properties of, 119
  cool melon summer soup, 119
  pure sunshine summer smoothie, 134

hip isolations, in belly dancing, 174–175

holy basil essential oil
  basil, maca, and sunflower summer
    exfoliating powder, 153
  beneficial properties of, 153, 158
  summer soak, 164
  sunflower shea summer oil, 158

home, peace in, 99

honesty and trust, as human needs, 30

honeydew melon
  birth of cool melon summer soup, 119
  pure sunshine summer smoothie, 134

hot lemon all-season water, 145

hummingbird spirit animal, 194

humor, sense of, as human need, 29

hydration, 11, 63, 68–69

I

in between state of consciousness, 97
  Yoga Nidra and, 183–185

individuation, 32

inner beauty, 8

inner child, 28

inner life
  design of, 52, 55–59
  reading set for, 83

inner temple, vision of one's, 57–58

internal narrative, rewriting one's, 53–54

interpersonal relationships, enlightenment
  and, 19

Iyengar, B. K. S., 167

J

jasmine essential oil
  beneficial properties of, 162
  jasmine lemon spring mist, 162

jazz, musical recommendations for, 201

Jerusalem artichokes
  beneficial properties of, 126
  goodness in a glass summer juice, 126

journals
  gratitude, 66
  self-symposium, 82

joy, breath of joy, 178

joyful living, 8, 41

joyfulness, as human need, 29

"joyous," 198

juices, 123–129
  all-season glorious greens, 129
  goodness in a glass summer juice, 126
  radiant immunity sour spring juice, 125
  slow-aging bitters winter juice, 123
  tastes like apple pie fall compote, 126

Jung, Carl, 190, 195

K

Kabbalah, 58

kale
  beneficial properties of, 32
  good fortune spring smoothie, 133

Kilbourne, Jean, 51

kintsigu, 20, 59, 87

knowing, as human need, 26

Kook, Abraham Isaac, 95, 186, 188

L

language, choosing one's own, 196–199

laughter and tears, as human needs,
  29–30

lavender
  beneficial properties of, 109
  lavender, matcha, and avocado oil
    spring exfoliating powder, 150
  pure poetry spring team, 109

learning, as human need, 26

Legs Up the Wall Pose, 183

lemon
  beneficial properties of, 125, 141, 145
  garlic-lemon drop winter water, 141
  jasmine lemon spring mist, 162
  radiant immunity sour spring juice, 125
  turmeric orange fall water, 145

lemon balm essential oil, pomegranate
  and melissa oil dense fall scrub, 154

lemon essential oil
  beneficial properties of, 157
  jasmine lemon spring mist, 162
  lemon primrose spring oil, 157

lemongrass essential oil, winter soak, 164

lemon primrose essential oil
  beneficial properties of, 157
  lemon primrose spring oil, 157

light rituals
  first light, 61
  solar light, 64
  third light, 66

light therapy, 11

ACKNOWLEDGMENTS

My heartfelt thanks to the Running Press team: Cindy De La Hoz, Kristin Kiser, Susan Van Horn, Katie Hubbard, Seta Zink, and Amber Morris, all of whom are an absolute dream to work with. So much gratitude to Coleen O'Shea who, over the course of over many years, patiently encouraged me to write this book, and to Nikki Van Noy, who made the process seamless, painless, and joyful. Thank you also to Amy Stanton for believing in me.

To my husband, Ran, and my children, Xandi and Olivia, who gave me the space and love to write this book, and make a lifelong dream come true. I am grateful to my dear friends for their kindness and understanding.

To my mom for her steadfast presence, my brother who always makes me laugh, and to my dad for being my dad.

And to life—all of it.

NOTES

SLOW BEAUTY